Understanding Your Body

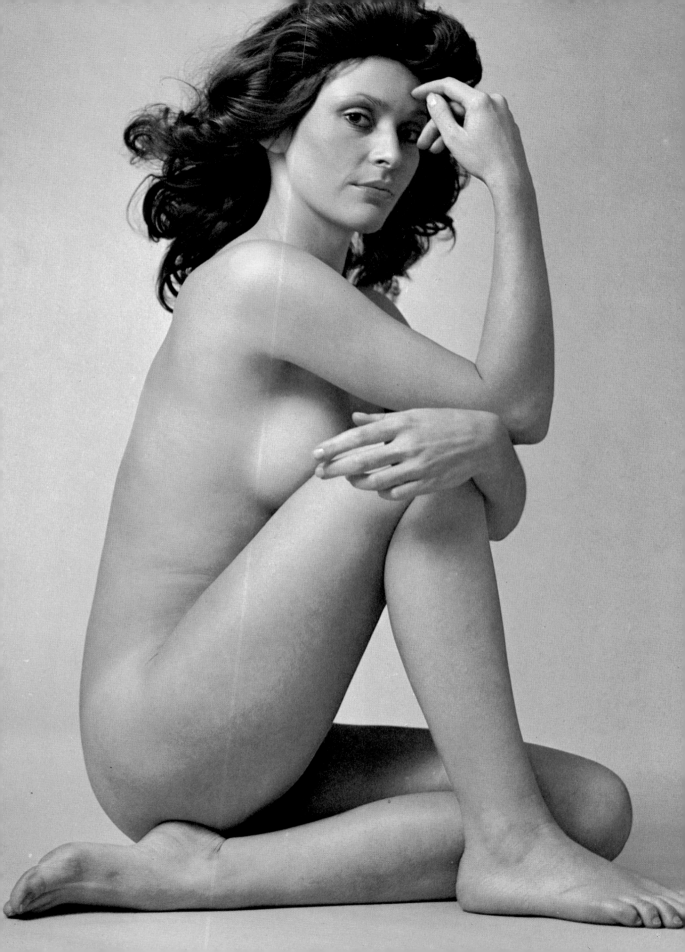

WOMAN ALIVE

Understanding Your Body

by Frederic C. Appel

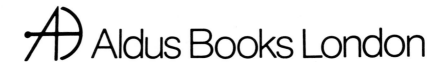 Aldus Books London

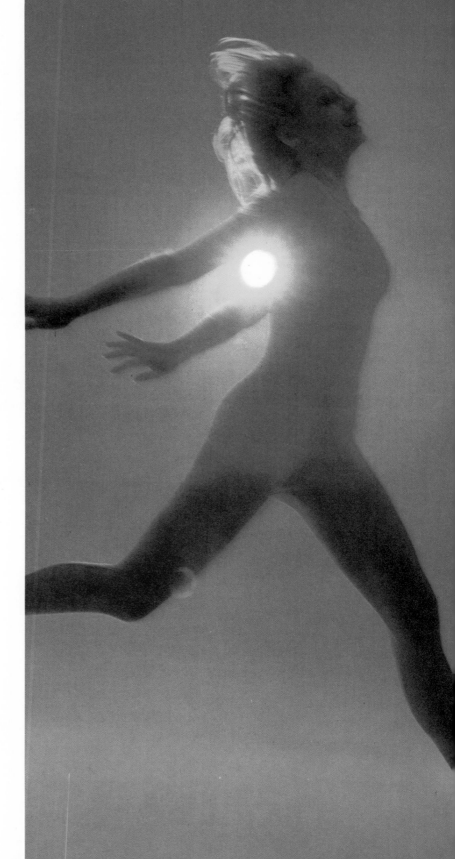

Series Coordinator: John Mason
Design Director: Guenther Radtke
Picture Editor: Peter Cook
Editor: Mary Senechal
Copy Editor: Mitzi Bales
Research: Elizabeth Lake
        Lynette Trotter
        Sarah Waters
Consultants: Beppie Harrison
           Jo Sandilands

Contents

This book is about health. Your good health. It starts with a clear and simple explanation of how the female body works, telling you just what you need to know about your own body in order to keep it in perfect condition. Later chapters lead you to proper care of yourself to make you feel on top of the world mentally and emotionally as well as physically. Here are facts about a woman's psychological outlook, about the nervous system, menstruation, and the right eating habits. A final section answers some often-asked questions on such important topics as aging, menopause, and sleep. In all, this book is a guide to the kind of vital health that makes you feel — and look — your best as today's Woman Alive.

A Woman's Body

This is a good time to be alive. Every day brings us new insights into the workings of the human body. And understanding the body is the key to health. But to people of past ages the body long remained a mystery. **Below:** the artist of 30,000 years ago emphasized woman's role as the giver of life.

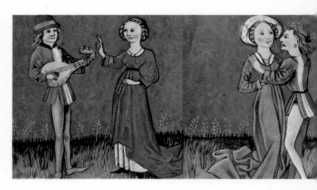

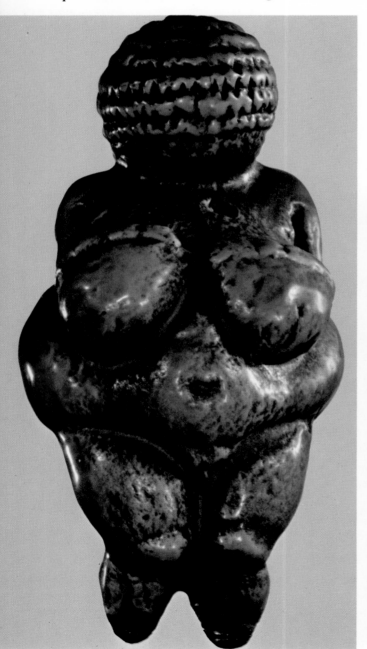

Above: the four moods of man. Doctors of the 1300's thought that the body held four "humors." The dominant humor determined temperament: sad, cheerful, violent, or lazy.

Below: in the 1200's surgical operations were rare. With little practical knowledge to go on, anatomists sometimes sketched the right organs—but often in the wrong places.

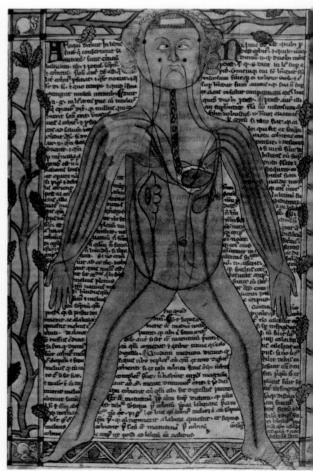

MS. ASHMOLE 399, FOLIO 19

6

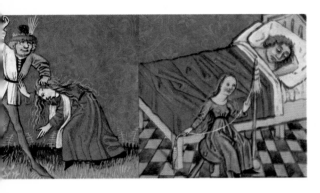

Below: learning how our bodies work is now an essential part of education. By studying a see-through model of a woman's body, these children will learn with ease lessons that baffled scientists for hundreds of years. Anatomy is no longer a puzzle. And while scientists continue to probe the secrets of the human body, modern medicine can already promise us longer and healthier lives than our ancestors dreamed could be possible.

Below left: the sperm held a completely formed embryo, according to biologists of the 1600's. The woman's body was merely the house in which the baby would grow.

Below right: the Italian artist Leonardo da Vinci made some of the first anatomical drawings of a woman's body. But his discoveries went unheeded for many centuries.

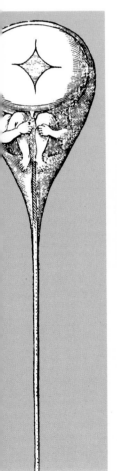

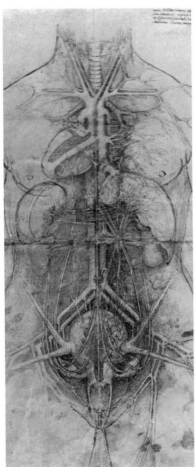

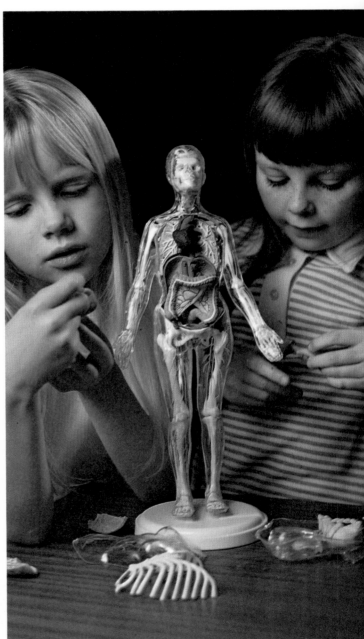

How We Abuse Our Bodies

Fashion and custom have often made women do weird and dangerous things to their bodies. Although fewer physical abuses exist today, drugs, drink, and gluttony still take a toll.

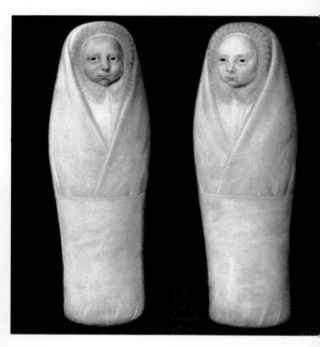

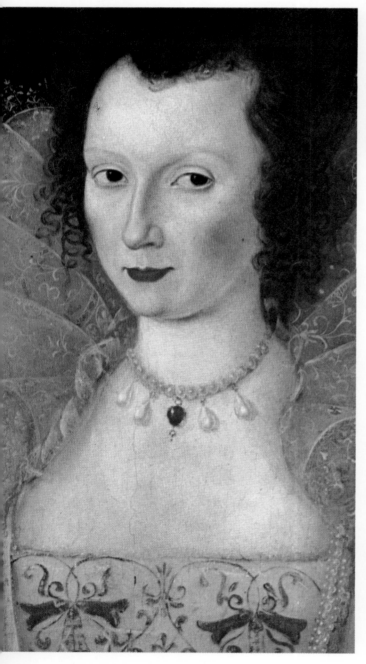

Above: babies were once wrapped in tight swaddling clothes to keep out "bad air."

Left: Elizabethan ladies wore poisonous cosmetics that actually ate away the skin.

Below: fashion in the 1830's demanded a tiny waist achieved by extremely tight lacing. This sometimes made women faint away.

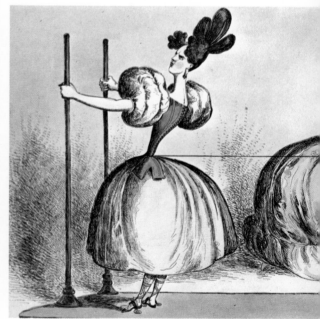

Below left: women of the Burmese Padaung tribe still wear heavy brass collars to stretch their necks. Built up as a girl grows up, these collars are never removed throughout life.

Below right: the desirable shape of 1909. Corsets like these were often so tight that they damaged the rib-cage and even forced vital organs dangerously out of shape.

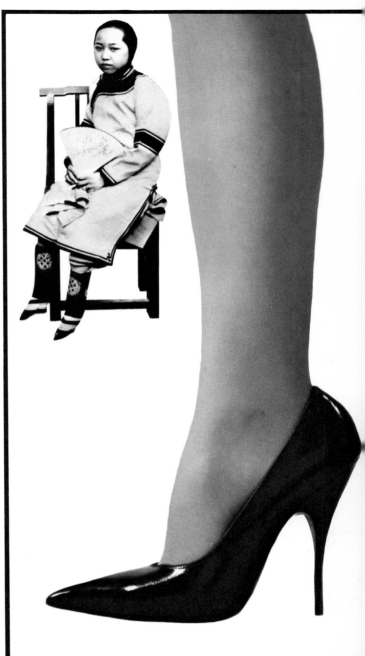

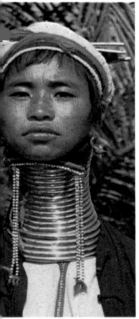

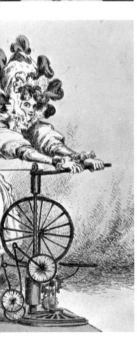

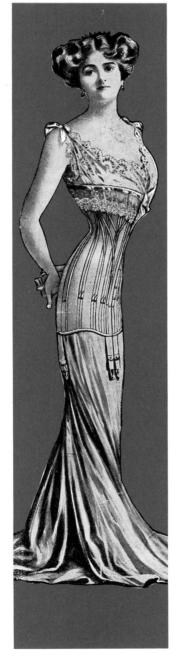

Above left: Chinese girls used to have their feet tightly bound from babyhood to stop them growing. Their bones became twisted, and walking was both difficult and painful.

Above: shoes like this are harmful, too. Apart from being uncomfortable to wear, they crush the feet, destroy natural balance, and make it hard to walk or stand.

Below: the plump woman in Frans Hals' famous 17th-century oil painting, *The Merry Company*, looks like she has already indulged heavily in the sausages and bread heaped high on the table. The habit of overeating is a hard one to break, as shown by current statistics on the number of people who are overweight or obese. Yet many continue to eat far more than they need for health.

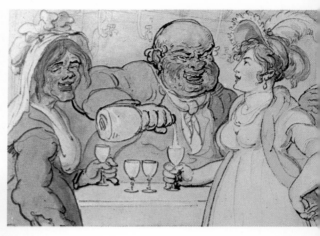

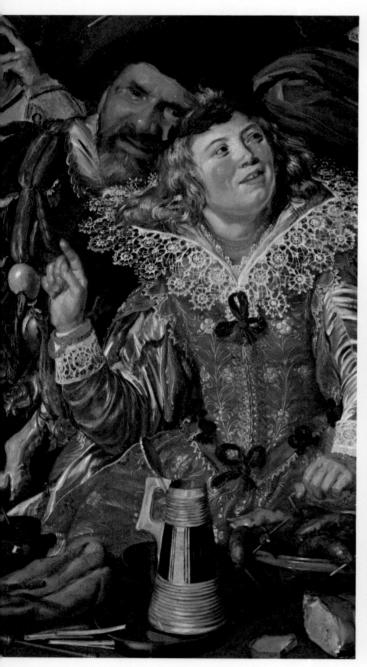

Above: how long before overdrinking makes the ravishing young woman look like the ravaged old woman? This drawing of the 1800's shows the evils of too much gin.

Below: sipping cola from a straw may be fun, but too much is far from good for children. Cola can become addictive.

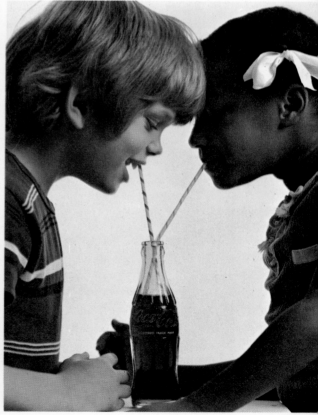

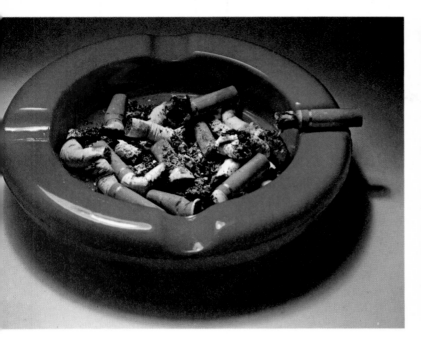

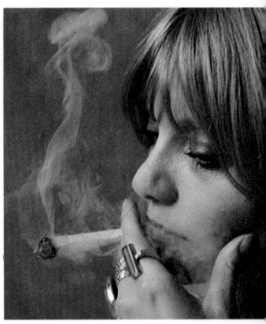

Above: the ashtray chockablock with cigarette stubs tells of a heavy smoker—someone who is running serious risk of getting lung cancer. Death statistics include a higher percentage of women each year.

Above right: many people today seek an escape from the pressures of life by smoking marijuana, even though its use is illegal.

Below: traffic, crowds, noise, and dirt—all are typical of New York and other big cities. The traffic and crowds add greatly to the stress and tension of modern city living. Noise has been proven to cause excess fatigue and insomnia. And dirt helps aggravate air pollution. Many women today do volunteer work with organizations that are trying to save and improve the natural environment.

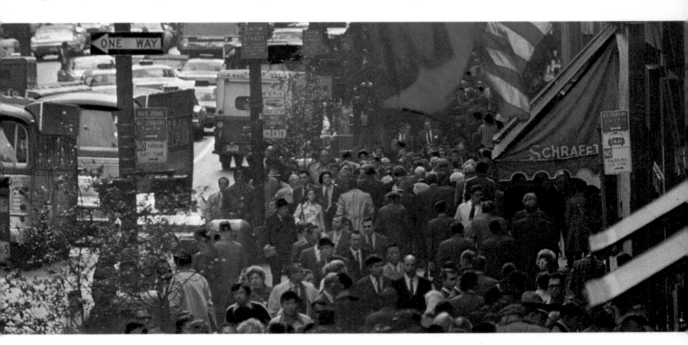

Copper Bracelets and other Cure Alls

Potions, brews, and cures are all part of a folk medicine that has been passed from generation to generation. Today, many traditional remedies are still known and used.

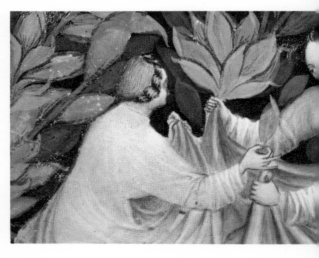

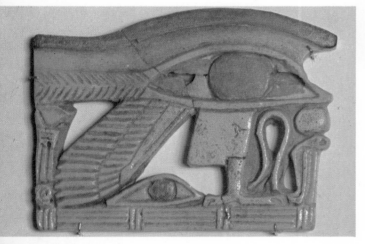

Above: the garden yields its sage to the women shown in a 15th-century miniature. Herbs have long been used medicinally.

Left and below left: ancient Egyptians made amulets, or good luck charms, to ward off sickness. People today sometimes wear copper bracelets as a preventative against rheumatism, or even as a cure.

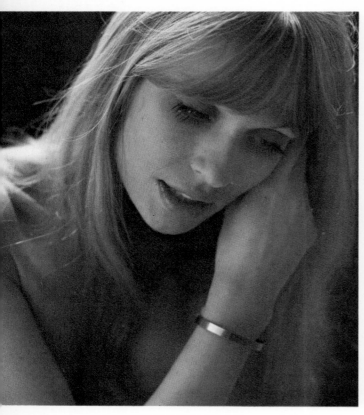

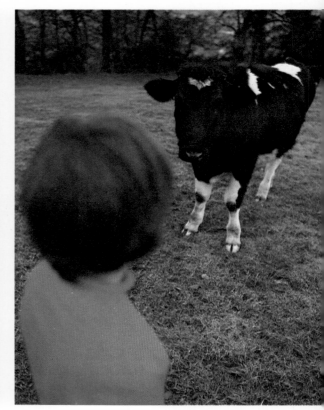

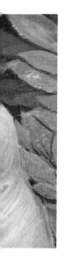

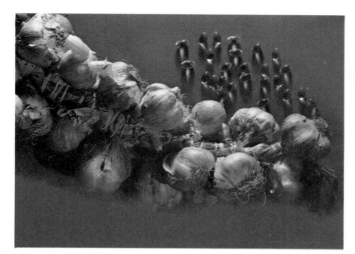

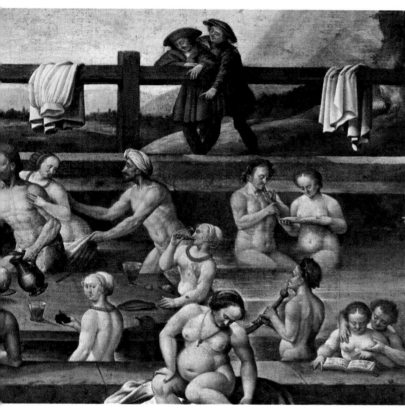

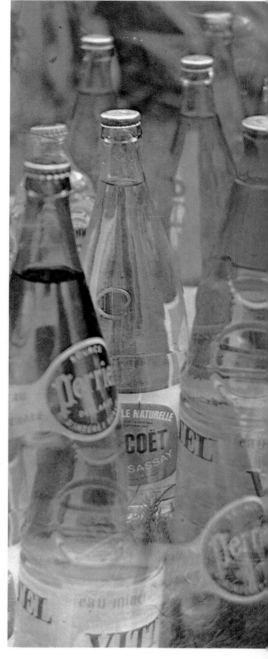

Above: "taking the waters" was the thing to do in the old days, and there still are some frequented mineral spas in the world. But the goings on, shown in this 16th-century painting, are hardly typical of today.

Left: boy eyes cow. Maybe he's heard the old tale that the breath of a cow cures whooping cough, and wants to see Bossy play doctor.

Top center: garlic not only enhances flavor of food, but is also said to aid health by stimulating appetite and digestion, clearing the head, and relieving coughs. Garlic now also comes in an easy-to-use capsule form.

Above right: bottled mineral waters, drunk on their own or with meals, are popular on continental Europe as an aid to digestion.

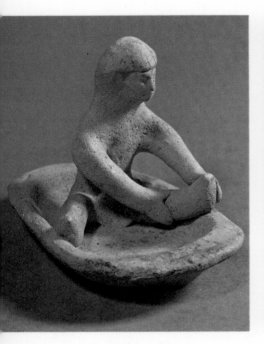

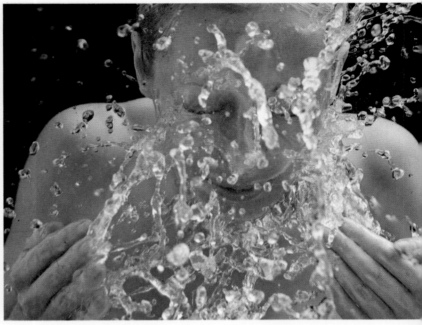

Health and Beauty

Happily for the modern woman, she is most often judged for the vitality, poise, and attractiveness that comes from simple good health and proper grooming. For her, beauty is the fruit of the bloom of health—and she can measure up just by common-sense care.

Above and above left: a splash of water is a fun way to start face care. Phoenician women of antiquity also bathed for beauty, as shown by this ancient terra cotta figurine.

Below left and below: when swimming started in Europe in the 1800's, women were swathed from neck to toe for modesty. Today, nothing need stand between you and the sun.

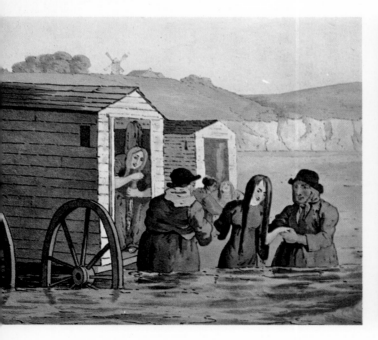

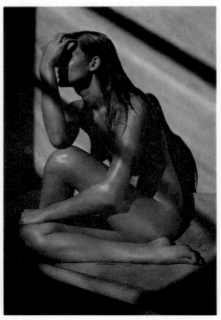

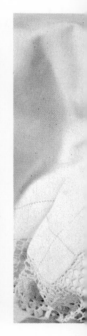

14

Below: the mouth-filling taste of a crisp apple is a treat that has a health bonus. Apples not only provide you with valuable vitamins, but also help keep teeth cleaner.

Bottom: "beauty sleep" and "sweet dreams" may be clichés, but restful and adequate sleep is essential to good looks—and a proper sleep is one that is filled with dreams.

Below: dressed comfortably for the season and wearing the right shoes, you could probably walk for miles. And what a world of good it would do you! Walking keeps you fit and trim, tones up muscles, and fights tension. A long ramble with your child can be filled with fun, a sense of adventure, and healthful exercise. Walking is also fun on your own, if you can get away by yourself.

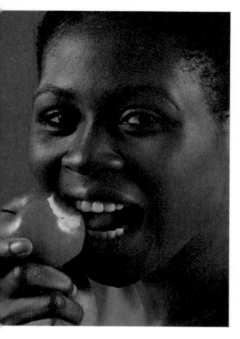

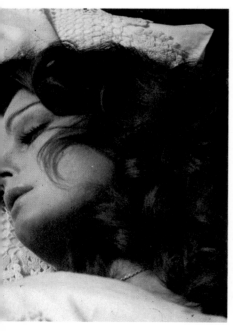

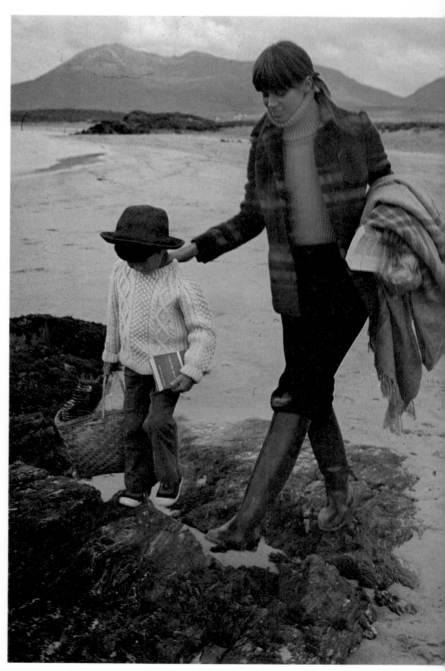

The Rhythm of Your Life

1

Since this is a book about health, let's start at the beginning. How do you feel? Right now, this very minute? Would you say you're in the pink of condition? Buoyant, sunny-natured, and up to most any challenge? Or perhaps you feel a bit off your peak, a trifle heavy and dull. Maybe you are even downright edgy and irritable.

However you feel, chances are that the present state of your body and emotions has something—possibly quite a bit—to do with your menstrual month. For, although countless outside pressures contribute to the way you feel at any particular moment, it is an established fact that your sense of well-being —the state of body and mind that we call health—is profoundly influenced by the fact that, in nature's eyes, your body was designed for childbearing. Whether you ever fulfill this biological role or not, your body has been provided with special organs and special functions. And, beginning with the time you reach puberty, your body prepares itself each month to bear a child. With nearly clockwork regularity, interrupted only by pregnancy, stress or illness, your womb builds up a special lining rich in tiny blood vessels to receive, nourish and protect a newly conceived baby. And if you do not become pregnant, the lining is broken down and shed each month in a flow of blood.

Every woman knows that there are days when, in spite of all life's problems, it feels good to be alive, when things run smoothly, and she feels in full control of her life. On the other hand, there are days—usually just before your period—when the outlook seems unbelievably gloomy. The whole world seems to be against you. And as if this weren't

Right: under the surface of a woman's everyday life, the menstrual cycle —which usually lasts for more than 30 years— moves in regular rhythm.

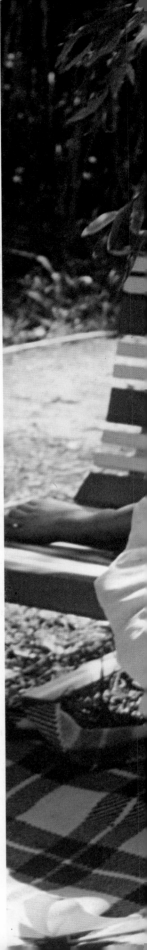

16

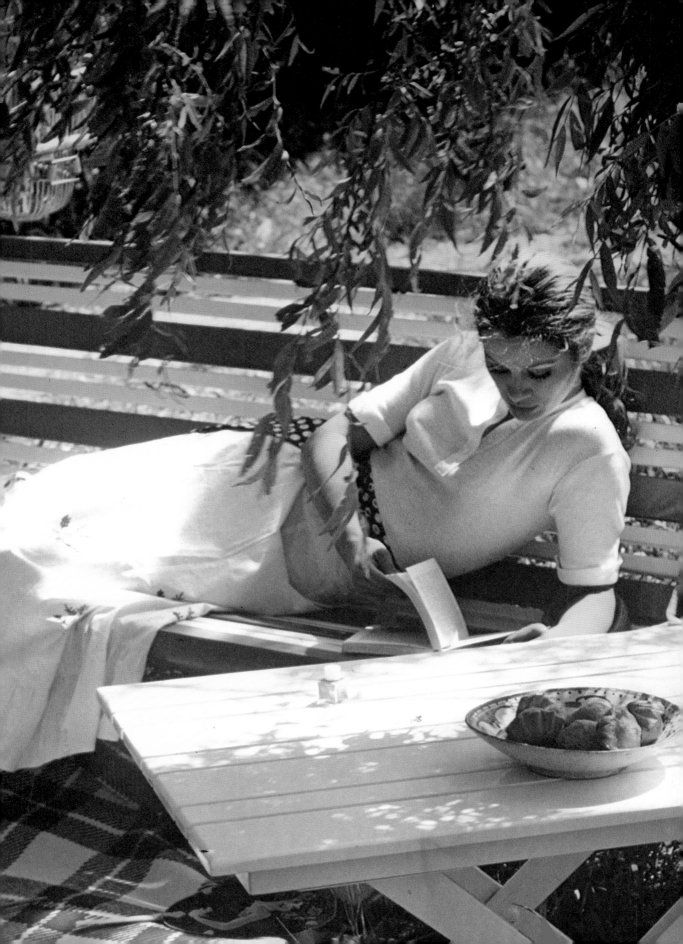

enough, you may be physically uncomfortable, too. Your abdomen may feel bloated and sore, and your breasts so tender that they hurt; your head aches, and you feel so tired that the least effort wears you out. Then, when your period begins, the dreary round of symptoms that may have troubled you for a week, or ten days, or more, somehow disappear as inexplicably as they came. You may not be dramatically filled with sweetness and light, but you certainly feel a great deal better.

It is only natural to think that when you are feeling good, you are normal, and when you are down in the dumps, you are "not yourself." In actual fact, however, both your ups and downs are characteristic of phases in your menstrual cycle, which runs from the beginning of one period to the first day of the next.

But what actually causes the bleeding to begin? Why does it stop? Why does it sometimes fail to appear on schedule even when you are not pregnant? And, most importantly, how can the natural process of menstruation have such a profound effect on the way women feel?

The answer to all these questions is tied very closely to the complex functioning of two walnut-sized organs located deep inside your abdomen. These are the ovaries—the glands of womanhood. Until about 50 years ago, physicians believed that the only job of the ovaries was to store egg cells and release one of them every 28 days or so throughout a woman's reproductive life. By 1923, however, scientists had discovered that the ovaries also function as chemical factories, manufacturing powerful, body-regulating hormones

known as *female sex hormones*. For women everywhere, this discovery was one of the paramount medical events of the century. For the female sex hormones are the key to your womanhood. It is they which swelled your breasts; gave your voice its womanly timbre; energized your mind and emotions. It is they which control your monthly periods and determine when you will have your menopause. And it is they which set in motion the physical and emotional seesaw on which every woman lives from one month to the next.

Before we see how these female hormones function, we need to take a brief look at how a woman's intimate anatomy is constructed and what the essential parts are called.

In contrast to men, whose sexual anatomy is almost completely external, the only part of a woman's sexual organs which can be seen on the outside of her body is the *vulva*. This is the name used by doctors to describe the whole area surrounding the opening of the *vagina*. It consists of two folds of flesh known as the larger lips *(labia majora)*, which are covered on the outside by pubic hair and kept moistened on the inside by special glands. Within the protective folds of the larger lips are the more delicate lesser lips *(labia minora)*, the opening of the vagina, the *urethra* (the opening from the bladder), and a small muscular and nerve-rich organ, the *clitoris*. This small organ, which is covered by a tiny fold of the lesser lips, is the female equivalent of the male penis. It lies in the upper part of the vulva above the urethra and the vagina. It is extremely sensitive to the touch and during sexual excitement it becomes erect and firmer. Its high degree of

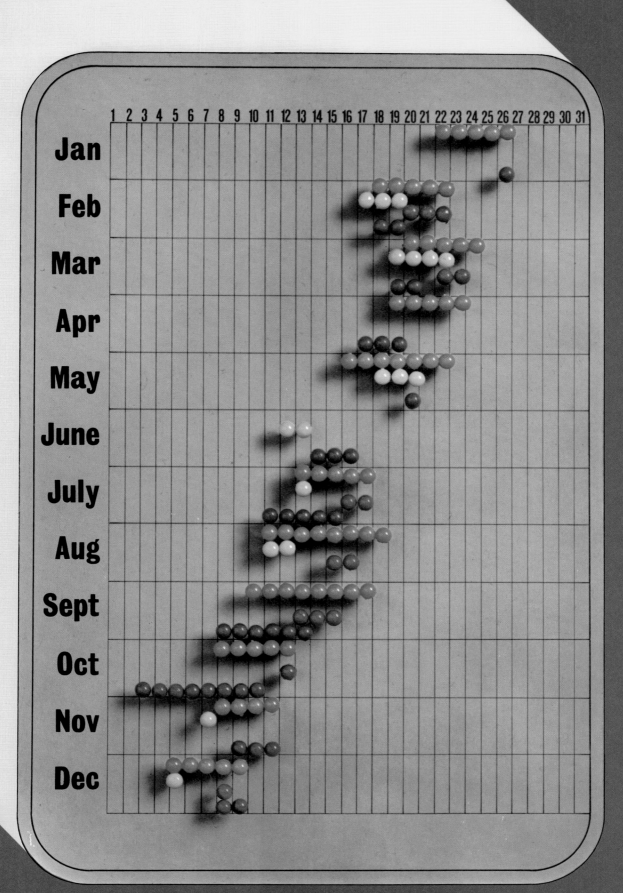

sensitivity is responsible for a good measure—but not all—of a woman's pleasure during intercourse.

A woman's external and internal sex organs are linked by the vagina, a muscular passage some three to four inches long. The vagina is strong, elastic, and extremely adaptable. Its task is to enfold the penis during intercourse, to receive sperm-carrying fluid, to serve as a canal through which a baby enters the world, and to carry out the menstrual flow during the monthly period.

The vagina leads to the *cervix,* the lower part of the womb, which extends into it. The cervix is yet another clue to the wonderful complexity of a woman's body. Normally about two inches long and the diameter of a quarter, the cervix virtually seals off the womb. Yet during labor this small muscular organ changes shape drastically and—without tearing or damage—stretches wide enough to let the baby pass from its prenatal home in the womb on the first stage of its journey into the outside world.

Womb is rather an old-fashioned word—more literary than scientific. Most doctors refer to this organ as the *uterus.* About the size and shape of a small pear with the narrower end pointing downward, the uterus lies deep within the body, between the bladder in front and the rectum behind, in a protective dish formed by your hip bones. Its function is to provide a safe haven in which the fertilized egg can be protected and nourished as it develops into a baby. During pregnancy, the complex system of muscles in the uterus enable it to stretch to accommodate the growing baby. The uterus is lined with a thin layer of tissue called the *endometrium.* It goes through many—almost daily —changes throughout the menstrual cycle.

The uterus communicates with the ovaries by means of the *Fallopian tubes.* These two small tubes hang from either side of the uterus, and the ovaries are loosely attached to them by a membranous sheet. At the upper ends of each of the Fallopain tubes, small, finger-like projections reach out to guide the

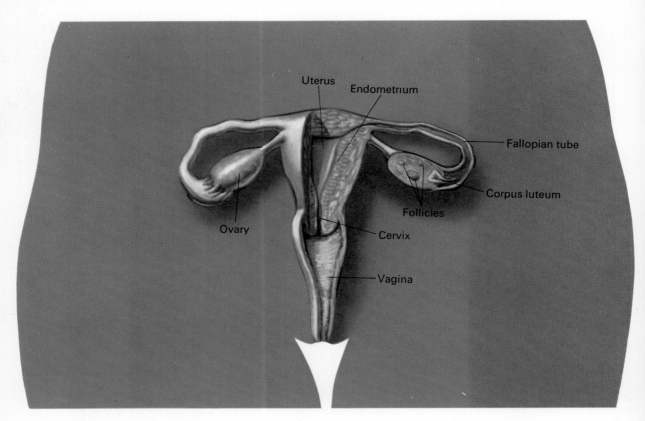

Right: the sex hormones, which have a profound effect on the way your body functions, are chemicals. Their important influence is simply a result of a series of chemical reactions, most of which are still imperfectly understood by the doctors of today.

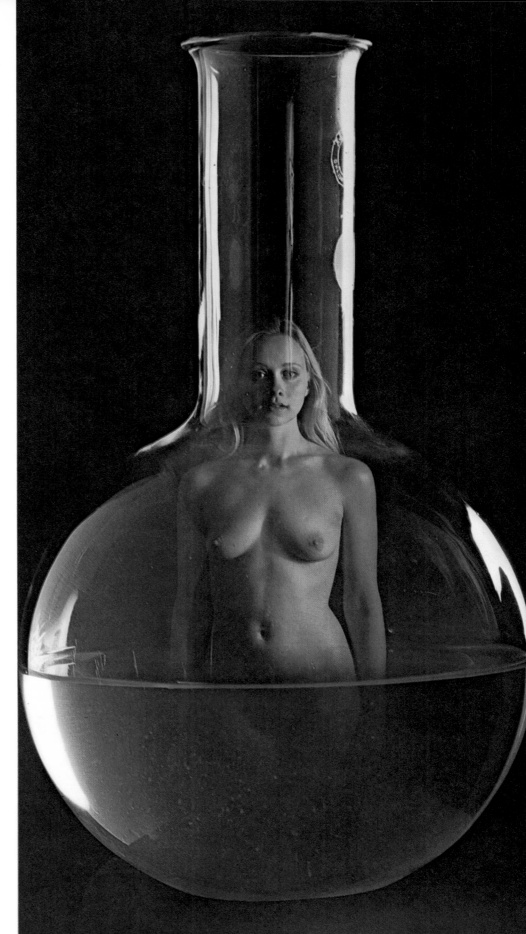

Left: the woman's reproductive organs are located deep inside her body as a protective measure. The vagina is the link between the internal and external sexual organs.

Right: four of the hormones that regulate the menstrual cycle are shown here as they influence your body. In orange is the FSH (follicle-stimulating hormone); in pink is the LH (luteinizing hormone); in yellow is the hormone estrogen; and in green is the hormone progesterone. When production of hormones falls off, a woman's menopause begins.

Below: the whole cycle of a woman's reproductive system is designed to produce new life and shelter the development of that new life within her body.

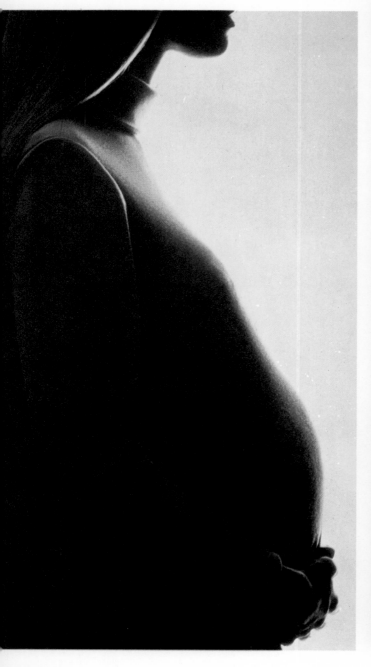

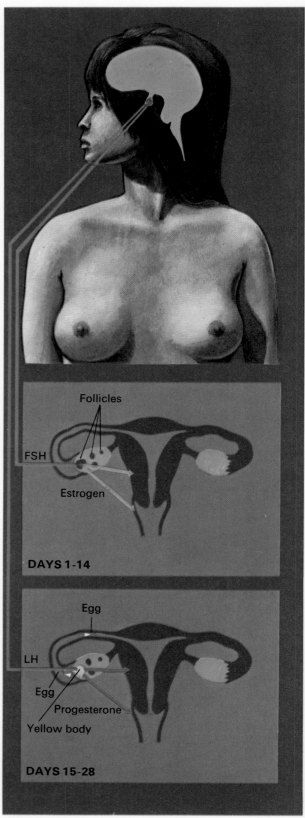

Follicles

FSH

Estrogen

DAYS 1-14

Egg

LH

Egg

Progesterone

Yellow body

DAYS 15-28

egg into an exceedingly small canal running down the tube's length. Once the egg has entered this canal, minute folds within the Fallopian tube move it downward on its way toward the uterus. And it is within the Fallopian tube that the sperm finds and unites with the egg to create new life.

The Fallopian tubes are thin because the egg they transport is no larger than a tiny dot, only just visible to the human eye. It is one of many thousands of eggs that have been inside your ovaries since before you were born. During your life, only a few hundred of these will ripen and mature to the stage where they can be fertilized to start the life of a new human being. Each egg is packaged in an envelope of special cells called the *follicle*. Your physical and emotional seesaw is set bobbing up and down by the chemical events taking place in the follicles as the eggs are ripened and cast free.

These events are not self-starting. They are powered by a master control panel in the brain called the *hypothalamus*, which is also in charge of many other vital bodily functions. The hypothalamus transmits the relevant signals to the *pituitary*—a small gland at the base of the brain—to time your menstrual rhythm.

The rhythmic pattern begins when your period starts. This is Day 1 of the cycle, when, in response to a command from the hypothalamus, the pituitary begins to secrete a chemical substance, or hormone, known as FSH (follicle-stimulating hormone). FSH acts as a kind of chemical messenger that flows through the bloodstream and signals to the ovary: "Begin to get an egg ready."

In answer to this signal, a number of egg follicles in the ovary begin to enlarge and also to produce the female hormone called *estrogen*. Estrogen production, which will continue for the first half of the cycle, causes the lining of the uterus to begin thickening in preparation for the arrival of a fertilized egg. During these 13 days or so, your feelings of well-being rise as the amount of estrogen in your blood increases.

Day 14, or thereabouts, is the day of

Now, as much as ever, the woman's body is meant for childbearing. But, with modern methods of birth control, the woman of today is free from the age-old fear and burden of an unwanted pregnancy. This gives her a meaningful choice in deciding when and if to have a family.

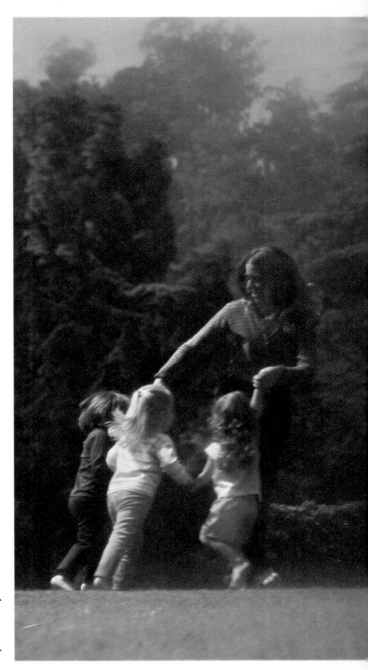

ovulation. Now the estrogen concentration in the blood is so high as to signal back to the pituitary: "Stop FSH production and begin to secrete luteinizing hormone (LH)." This hormone surges through the bloodstream to the ovary and causes the follicle nearest the surface to burst like a tiny balloon and release its egg into the finger-like ends of the Fallopian tube.

Some women know exactly when this happens because they feel the release of the egg as a pain on one side of the abdomen. The pain may be on the right side one month and the left side another month, depending on which ovary has released an egg. The pain occurs because, when the egg pops out of the follicle, a small amount of fluid or blood also escapes and may irritate the sensitive inside lining of the pelvic cavity. Normally the pain is mild and short lasting. The time of ovulation can also sometimes be determined by a rise in temperature. But it is usually extremely difficult to pinpoint the exact moment when ovulation occurs. Most women remain quite unaware that, deep inside their body, a little follicle, less than half in inch in diameter, has set free its tiny egg.

The egg has but a few hours to live—probably not more than 48, possibly only 12. It is during this short time that you can become pregnant. Sperm, however, have a longer life-span than the egg, and may remain active inside a woman's body for as long as four days. So, if you and your husband have intercourse on the days just before ovulation, it is possible that you will conceive. But, as you know, most months the egg is not fertilized, and it soon dies. The menstrual cycle, however, has been set in motion to prepare for a possible pregnancy, and it has to continue for two more weeks.

Ovulation is the high point of the menstrual cycle and often signals the peak of your own well-being, the time when you are likely to feel your best. But remember that the egg only lives for a brief period and, if you do not become pregnant, it is not long before the body flashes the change of signals that begins the second phase of your menstrual cycle, when your physical and emotional outlook may become less cheerful. Some women are almost immediately crushed with feelings of depression, fatigue, irritability, and physical discomfort; for others, the symptoms gradually creep up on them as the month progresses; still others feel almost no ill effects.

As soon as the egg has escaped, LH starts to turn the cells of the burst follicle yellow. The follicle—now known as the *yellow body*—is still concerned with caring for the egg that has left it. Now not only does it continue to secrete estrogen but it also begins to produce the second female hormone, *progesterone,* which causes further changes in the lining of the uterus, putting on the finishing touches needed for the well-being of the fertilized egg should it come to rest there. As Dr. Gifford Jones, a Canadian woman's specialist, puts it, "estrogen prepares a soft bed for a possible pregnancy (and) progesterone goes a step further by turning down the covers and slipping a hot water bottle between the blankets."

If you become pregnant, the yellow body steps up its hormone output to preserve the precious endometrial lining, and will continue to care for the baby for about 12 weeks.

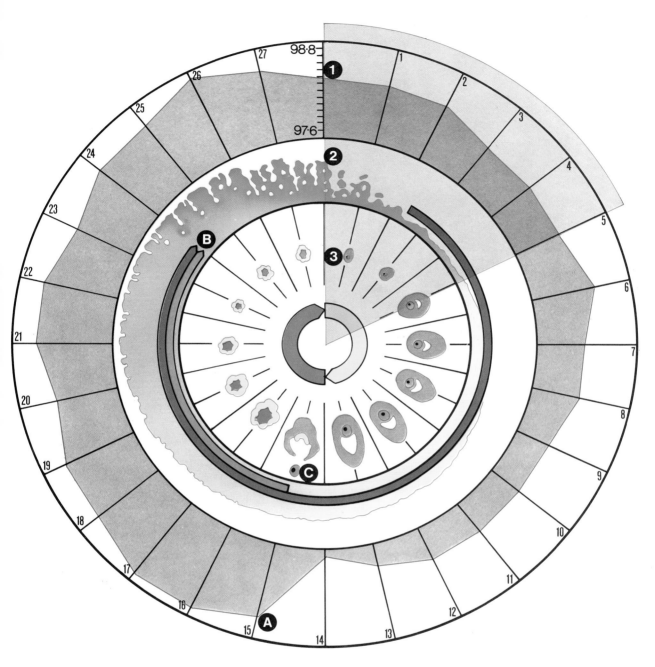

Above: a diagram of a menstrual cycle. The pie-shaped wedge in pink shows the actual period. The purple outline (1) shows the variation in body temperature. Notice the sharp rise at (A), just after ovulation. Changes in the uterine lining are shown starting at point (2). The olive green line is estrogen, which starts to build up the lining while the bleeding is still in progress. The light green line represents progesterone, which completes the preparation of the uterine wall. Its production starts on about day 14. When the level of these two hormones fall (B), the lining shrinks, and the top part breaks away. This starts the menstrual flow. Follicle development (3) begins when FSH, indicated by the yellow semicircle, causes several egg follicles to enlarge. LH, marked by the blue semicircle, is secreted about day 13. It causes one follicle to release an egg. That follicle then becomes a yellow body, from which progesterone is discharged to finish the buildup of the lining. It must be remembered that all these processes are constantly ongoing ones in the body.

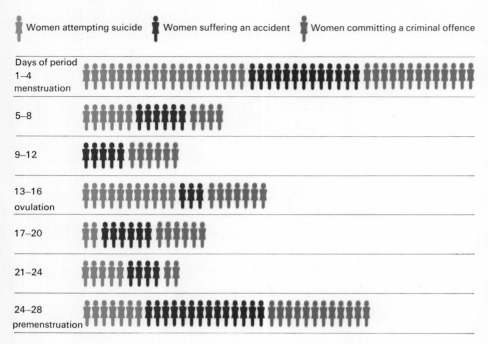

Women attempting suicide | Women suffering an accident | Women committing a criminal offence

Days of period
1–4 menstruation

5–8

9–12

13–16 ovulation

17–20

21–24

24–28 premenstruation

when hormones from the placenta and embryo take over control of the pregnancy. During this time, the hormone secreted by the yellow body will also inhibit further menstruation.

But when, as happens mostly, there is no baby to care for, the yellow body degenerates after 10 or 12 days, and the concentration of estrogen and progesterone in the blood falls off. This sharp decline in the flow of hormones signals to the uterus that this month's work has ended without pregnancy. The endometrial lining cannot be used again. It begins to shrink and, as it does so, it creases up tiny blood vessels within it. These provide blood to wash away the top part of the lining which has been built up so carefully during the preceding weeks. The uterus contracts to release the blood—and your period begins.

No sooner has the menstrual flow begun than your body's chemical clock rings the starting signal again. The lower part of the endometrial lining immediately starts to prepare a new one. In the ovaries, the follicles begin to swell and secrete a new flow of estrogen—and, as far as you're concerned, you should be feeling tops.

The ebb and flow of estrogen and progesterone is the basic rhythm of your life. And it is the fluctuating levels of these hormones

that play a vital part in determining your physical and emotional well-being during the menstrual cycle. This is because the ovaries that produce these hormones are just one part of a whole system of glands, called *endocrine glands,* which exert a major influence on every phase of human existence. Each of these glands is like a department in the intricate chemical factory of your body. Each one is busy producing hormones which ensure the proper harmonious functioning of the body factory as a whole. And they are all interrelated and linked by the bloodstream, which serves as the factory intercom system. A disturbance in any one of the endocrine glands can therefore cause changes in the others.

During the first half of your menstrual cycle, you can usually forget all about what your hormones are up to. At this time, your ovaries should be producing plenty of hormones in properly balanced quantities, and, barring the effects of outside stresses and strains, you are likely to feel as well as can be. But, during the second phase of the cycle, the level of hormones produced by the ovaries begins to fluctuate. And it is this variation that is thought to react with other body hormones to trigger off physical and

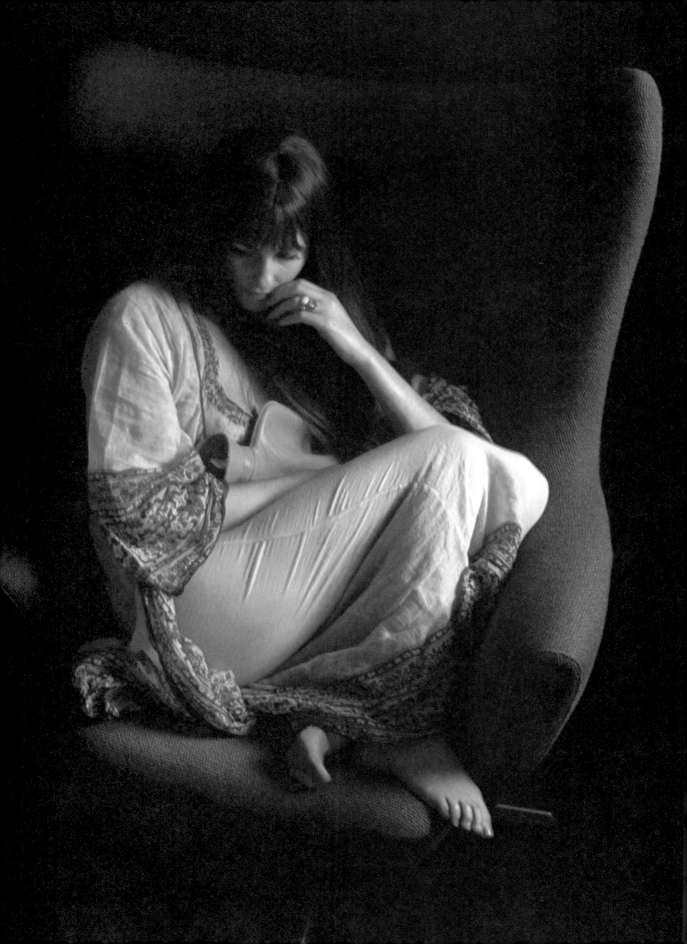

emotional changes that affect you so much.

Doctors group all these uncomfortable periodic disturbances under the name *premenstrual tension*, because they usually occur a few days before menstruation begins. But, as we have seen, premenstrual tension may come at any time from ovulation onward, and the symptoms may continue, on and off, during the next 14 days or so. Some women even feel at their worst during the first day or two of their period.

Just as the start of these physical and emotional changes varies, so do the kind and intensity of the symptoms—to such an extent that we may not always recognize them for what they are. And, to make matters even more complicated, most women have different symptoms from one month to the next.

Anxiety, depression, irritability, indecision and fatigue are perhaps the most characteristic symptoms that strike women just before menstruation. And research has shown that most of the accidents in the home occur during this phase of the menstrual cycle, that women drivers commit far more traffic violations then, and that as much as 93 per cent of female crimes are committed during the premenstrual phase.

Then there is that uncomfortable bloated sensation of which nearly all women complain. Before your period you may find that you weigh anything from 2 to over 10 pounds more than usual. Doctors agree that, for some reason or other, the body retains more fluid at this time of the month than at any other. It is this increased collection of fluids in the tissues that is generally believed to be responsible for the symptoms of heaviness, tender breasts, swollen legs and painful, prominent varicose veins. An increase of fluid in the cells of the brain might cause headaches; and in the skin, it can make for pimples and itching. The kind of symptom depends on where the fluid collects.

What can one do about premenstrual tension? Fortunately no woman suffers from all the possible premenstrual disturbances at the same time. Luckily, too, the symptoms are usually slight at first and only become troublesome just before the period. Most women manage, for their symptoms are relatively mild. Once a woman can relate her irritability, depression, fatigue, headaches, or whatever, to her menstrual cycle, and knows that, in a few days, she will be back to normal, she can often adapt herself emotionally to take her "low time" in her stride. But a little common sense planning can also be a great help. Try to save routine jobs for the time when you expect premenstrual symptoms, rather than undertaking some major project that requires a lot of energy or concentration.

In addition, doctors advise cutting down on fluid and salt intake during the days before your period. You don't need to limit the amount of salt you use in cooking, but try not to add more at the table, and drink no more than four cups of liquid a day. Smaller meals, but with plenty of protein, can help, and so can in-between snacks of fruit or cheese.

For those who have great discomfort, a visit to the doctor is the answer. He may not be able to correct the hormonal imbalance which is at the bottom of the trouble, but he can prescribe treatment to take care of the symptoms. For example, he may give you drugs called "diuretics" to stimulate your kidneys and rid you of that bloated feeling. And if you have several symptoms at once, he can often prescribe a drug that will dispose of them all in one go. In many cases, the contraceptive pill is also found to be very effective in abolishing premenstrual symptoms. So if premenstrual tension is a real problem for you, don't hesitate to seek medical advice. After all, even 4 or 5 days spoiled by premenstrual tension is too much, and you ought to do something about it.

Up to now, we have been talking about the menstrual cycle as if it were an absolutely regular series of events. Your own experience will tell you that this isn't the case at all. And most doctors will say that there is no need to worry if you find that you don't

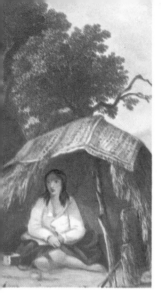

The fact that healthy women bleed at regular intervals has been regarded with fear and awe in most societies. Above: like many other primitives, American Indians kept menstruating women in isolation. Below: the monthly period was an unmentionable curse to Victorians. Right: today, periods do not restrict activity.

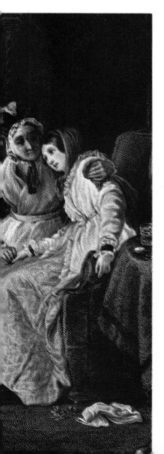

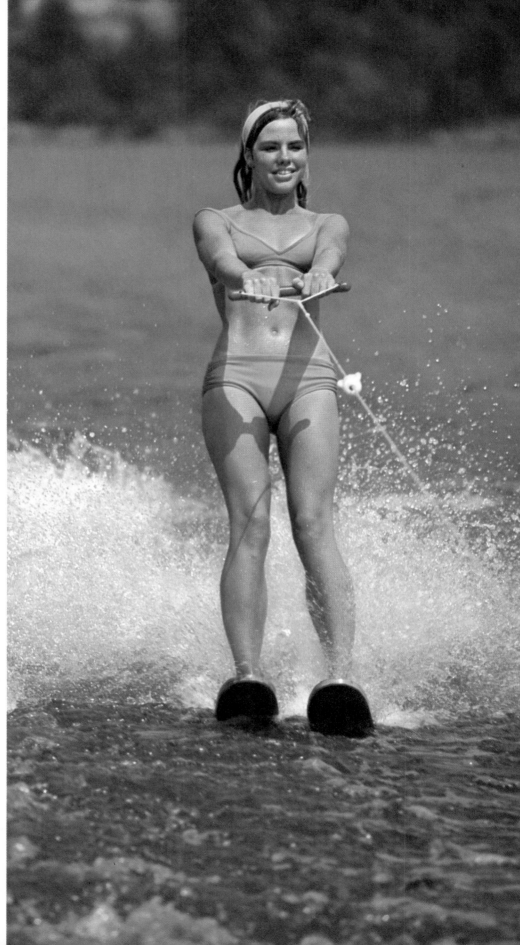

menstruate every 28 days on the dot.

It may be perfectly normal to have your period every 21 days, every 35 days, or any time in between. Sometimes the cycle may be even shorter or longer than that. No two women are exactly alike in this. You have your own personal timing, and this, too, is subject to a certain amount of individual variation. So, if your period varies from the supposed norm—but is regular, within a few days, for you—there is nothing to be concerned about. If you do worry, follow the sensible practice of consulting your doctor.

Just as the timing of the menstrual cycle varies from one woman to another, so does the duration of the period. A period usually lasts from 3 to 5 days, but it may last for only 1 or 2 days, or continue for 6, 7, or even 9 days. A long cycle may result in a heavier flow. But this is not always the case, and if your period is late, there is no need to dread having an extra heavy one. Although an average flow amounts to no more than three or four tablespoons, it can often be scantier or more profuse. It is hardly surprising, then, that doctors say the only regular thing about menstruation is its variability.

The important thing to note is that any change in your own personal rhythm (if you usually have 28-day cycles and suddenly begin having 21-day cycles, for example) requires looking into. In the same way, much heavier bleeding than usual during your period, an increase in the length of your periods, bleeding between periods, or missed periods, should all be checked.

Don't immediately jump to the conclusion that these variations have some dreadful significance. They can be the result of one, or several, of an amazing number of factors, both physical and emotional. Worry, for instance, is often at the root of the trouble. A dread of becoming pregnant, or a strong desire to conceive, may delay a period. Moving, changing your job, taking exams, having a quarrel with your husband or boyfriend, being concerned over a child's illness, all can disturb your menstrual rhythm. Changes of climate or environment

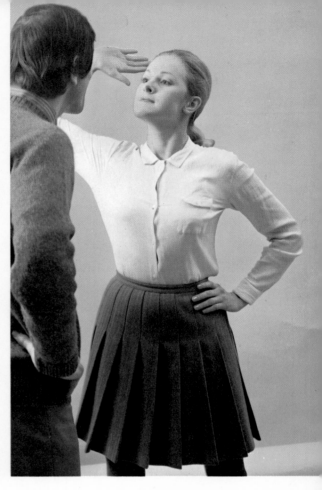

The close connection between emotions and body is obvious when a trivial quarrel upsets your monthly rhythm, delaying or accelerating your period.

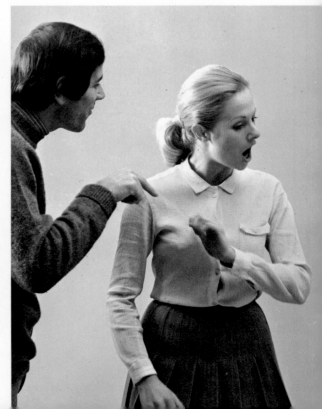

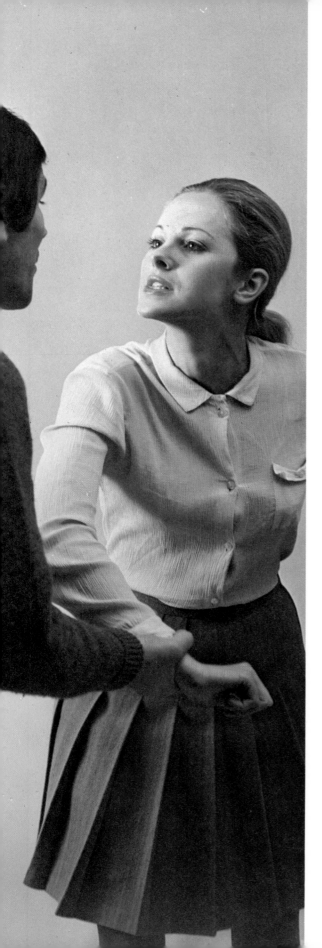

can bring on your period (even if the previous one only ended a few days before), or delay it, make it exceptionally short or annoyingly long. Illness—even a common cold—can make a period early or late, and a badly balanced diet can often cause missed periods.

But, just in case a change in your period pattern signals some physical problem, it is obviously better to check with your doctor. And since worry is a prime cause of irregularity—and never did anyone any good anyway—the best course of action is obviously to seek an explanation of what's gone wrong. Sometimes that in itself is enough to set things straight again.

Menstruation is part and parcel of good physical and mental health. As we have already seen, the menstrual cycle has only one function—to prepare the body for a possible pregnancy—and menstruation is no more than the natural shedding of the uterine lining when that pregnancy fails to happen. It has nothing to do with ridding the body of poisonous products, or "bad blood." In fact since menstrual blood is freshly made every few weeks, it is almost the newest blood in the body—just the opposite of bad blood. And this blood neither harms you if it doesn't come out, nor weakens you when it does.

Luckily today we know a great deal more about periods. Modern women have escaped from the sort of restrictions and beliefs that turned our female forbears into semi-invalids every menstrual period. But we still have to cope with a few superstitions and taboos inherited from less enlightened days. In the distant past, people believed that menstrual blood somehow prevented pregnancy, and was therefore a danger to all growing things. A woman who was having her period was kept apart from the community, for it was believed that she could stop crops from ripening, wither fruit or flowers, and turn wine or milk sour by her very presence. Ridiculous though all this may seem to us, these superstitions are still accepted in parts of the world today.

For every girl, the beginning of menstruation marks the beginning of womanhood. Even in our society, in which the first period goes unmarked by any ceremony, the event retains a special importance for a girl—and often for her mother too.

As time went on, it came to be believed that menstruation was not only dangerous but unclean and weakening, too. This gave rise to another batch of myths, some of which are still being passed on from mother to daughter. Certain foods, such as raspberries, are said to be "bad for you" if eaten during a period. Washing your hair during a period is thought by some to increase or stop the menstrual flow, cause a cold, or even pneumonia. A permanent wave is said not to take, a filling in a tooth will not last. It is said to be dangerous to take a bath, or do any exercises at this time.

Of course, there is no truth whatsoever in any of these beliefs. There is no reason at all to change your normal routine during a period. You can go to the hairdresser, bathe or shower, walk or swim, or dance all night, if you feel you want to.

"That's all very well," you might say, "but if menstruation is so normal, why do some women have such painful periods?" Unfortunately no one knows for certain what causes these unpleasant monthly cramps, but modern research indicates that they may be the result of the uterus contracting spasmodically, instead of rhythmically, just before and at the start of a period. Psychological factors also play their part, and the girl whose mother has warned her to expect painful periods is almost certain to suffer from menstrual cramps. Although a doctor must decide what treatment is needed in each individual case, hormone treatment is often effective in severe cases in which there is nothing physically wrong. This usually takes the form of the contraceptive pill, which acts by making the

pituitary "think" that the body has enough estrogen and progesterone (as if the woman were pregnant), so that it stops production of FSH and LH, and no eggs are released from the ovary. The period will then usually be painless.

Pain and tension seem rarely to go together. Those who have painful periods usually do not suffer from premenstrual tension. Conversely, those who have premenstrual tension usually have little or no pain during their periods. It also goes by age. Painful periods occur most often up to the age of 25, and premenstrual tension after that.

What about when your reproductive life comes to a close? Having seen the vital role that the female hormones play in the menstrual cycle, it will hardly come as a surprise to learn that the menopause occurs when your body stops production of estrogen and progesterone. Nowadays, however, just as modern medicine can take care of menstrual problems, it can also combat the troublesome symptoms of the menopause with the aid of hormone replacement drugs.

By this time you must have begun to feel that you are no more than a slave to nature's obsessive fixation on reproduction. Nothing could be further from the truth, for women today have the right—and available knowledge—to decide for themselves or with a loved one when, if ever, they shall have a baby. For the first time in history, a woman's social role can be separated from reproduction. Nevertheless, *you*—meaning the precious self which is largely mind and spirit—do live in a woman's body. The key to health lies in understanding it.

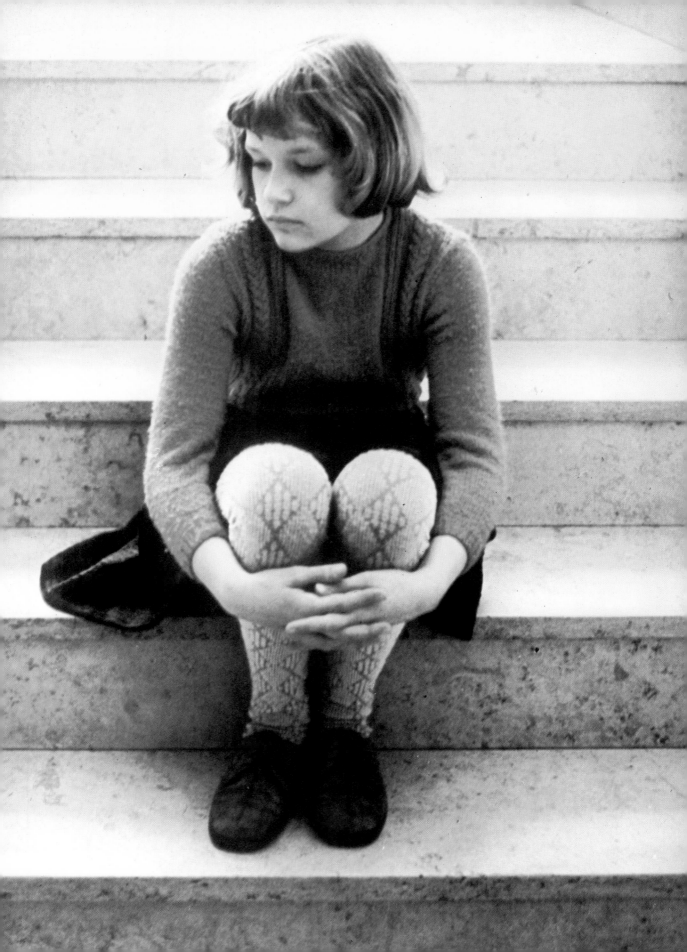

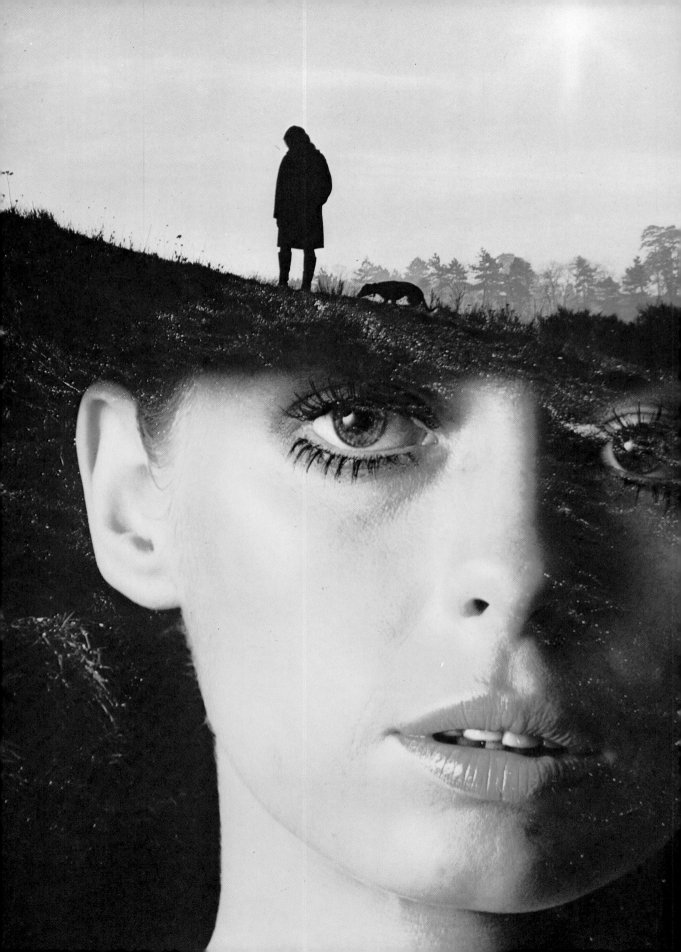

You and Your Brain

2

Your awareness of the world at any one time can be colored by your mind, filling in the present with the emotions of a dimly-remembered or repressed past experience.

We all worry. And anyone who has ever spent a sleepless night fretting over a problem, suffered from a nervous headache after an argument, developed a stomachache just before an exam, or felt an urgent desire to go to the bathroom at the start of an important occasion, knows how "nerves" can affect their health.

The body does not always react at once to emotional stresses and strains. Take the case of Shirley, a lively mother of three in her mid-thirties. For the past ten years her husband Ted had worked for a company in St. Louis. When Ted came home one day with the news that his boss wanted to transfer him to a much better paying job in the East, Shirley agreed right away that he should accept. She was delighted for him, but she had no idea how difficult the months ahead would be for her. Ted had to leave almost immediately to start his new job and find a new house for his family. Meanwhile, Shirley flung herself into the thousand and one details of moving. Between packing and planning, reassuring her children about the move, and saying goodbye to all her friends, Shirley had little time to think of herself.

Once in her new home, Shirley had to cope with a hectic round of unpacking, reorganizing, finding a school for the children, and adjusting to a whole new way of life. But after about six months, the whole family seemed to have settled down happily. Ted was doing well in his job, and the children had made new friends. Shirley had every reason to feel pleased with herself. But instead she felt run-down and depressed. She began to be plagued with persistent indigestion that kept her awake at night,

Viewed simply, your nervous system is a mass of pathways for conveying information to and from the brain. The sensory nerves carry messages from the body to the brain, and the motor nerves issue instructions from the brain to the voluntary and involuntary muscles of your body.

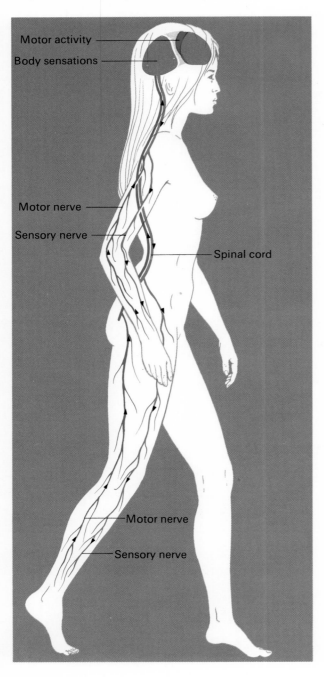

Motor activity

Body sensations

Motor nerve

Sensory nerve

Spinal cord

Motor nerve

Sensory nerve

prevented her from enjoying her meals, and made her feel generally miserable.

She couldn't figure out what was the matter with her, and was even more puzzled when her doctor declared that there was nothing physically wrong. When he asked if anything was worrying her, Shirley told him, quite truthfully, that everything was fine for her and her family. "But think back over the last twelve months or so," prompted the doctor. "Have you had any emotional upsets during that time?"

It was then that Shirley remembered how, through all the upheaval of the move, she she had kept her mind on the countless things she had to do and had not allowed herself to think of how much she resented leaving her old home and all her friends behind. She had worried about whether the children would settle down in new schools, whether her husband would like his new job, whether her elderly, widowed mother would manage so many miles away from her, and whether she herself would adapt to life in a strange city.

Shirley was suffering from a *psychosomatic* illness (from the words "psycho," meaning mind, and "soma," meaning body). Out of love for her husband, she had dismissed her apprehensions about the move from her mind. But those feelings did not disappear. They remained buried away in the back of her mind. And they continued to communicate, through her brain, with her nervous system, which eventually responded by producing unpleasant physical symptoms.

There are many such examples of the interaction between brain and body, of the effect of thought on the way we feel. And it is

For your brain, not all parts of the body are equally important in giving sensory information. Your face, hands, and feet do the outstanding work.

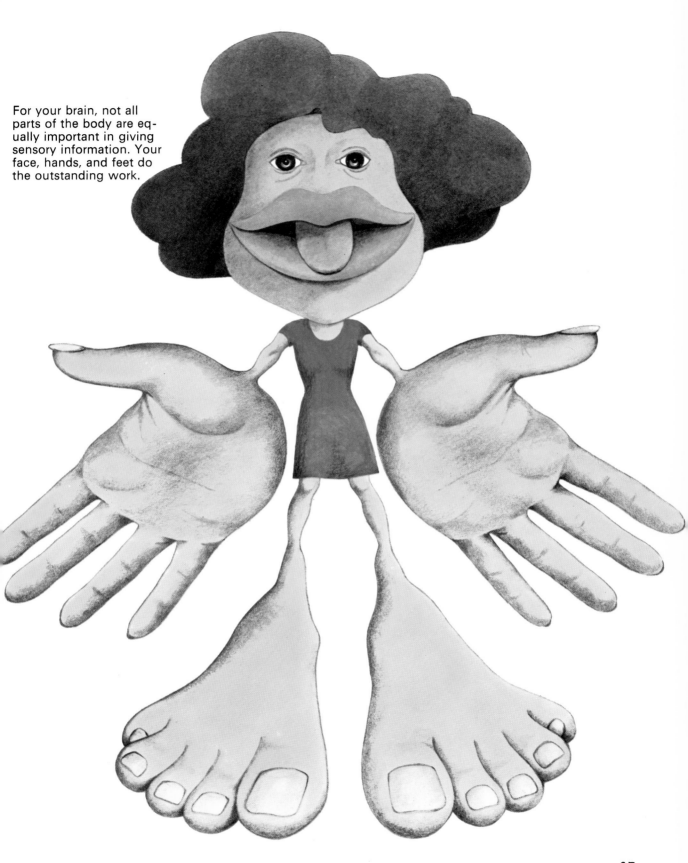

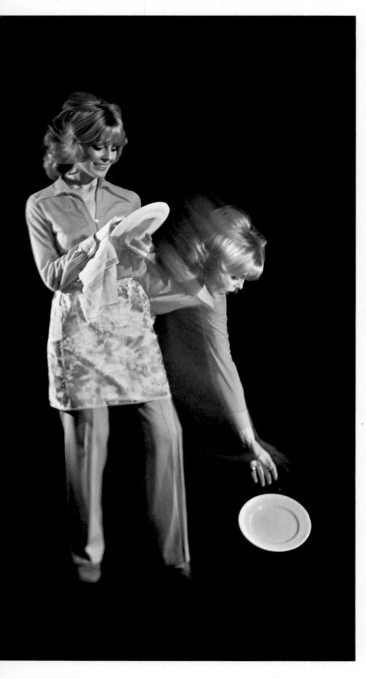

A swift flow of adrenalin, which supplies extra blood to your muscles for quicker action, helps you meet such a minor emergency as a falling plate.

vital for us to know something about this powerful relationship, so that we can put it to our own uses for the sake of good health and well-being.

Your brain is the seat of your entire world. Your eyes, nose, ears, tongue, and skin supply your brain with information about the world around you. And all that you *know* about your surroundings is derived from the way your brain interprets these signals from your senses.

And just as your brain keeps you in contact with the outside world, nothing goes on inside your body without your brain— although not necessarily your conscious mind—being aware of it. Every moment of your life, signals from the various parts of your body are being transmitted to the brain, which interprets these signals to tell you what is happening and how you feel.

Some feelings that seem to be located in other parts of your body are really created in your brain. One such example is sexual excitement and orgasm. The pioneering research of William Masters and Virginia Johnson in St. Louis, Missouri, indicates that, while a woman's orgasm originates with pleasurable stimulation of the clitoris and vagina, she may experience it as a complete involvement of the body. Orgasm apparently does not take place at all without the intervention of her brain. If a woman does not feel in the mood, no amount of physical contact of the type that produces sexual climax during intercourse will cause even mild sexual excitement. Only when her brain is tuned to sexual responsiveness can physical contacts produce orgasm.

Orgasm is only one of the body responses

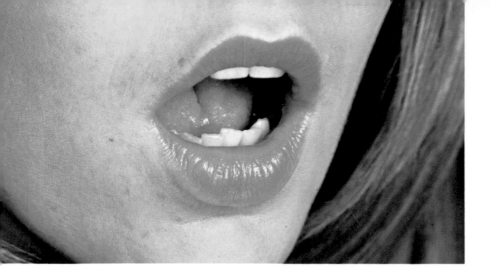

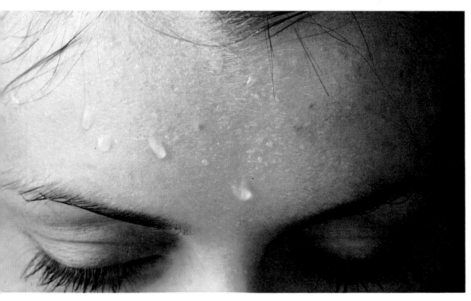

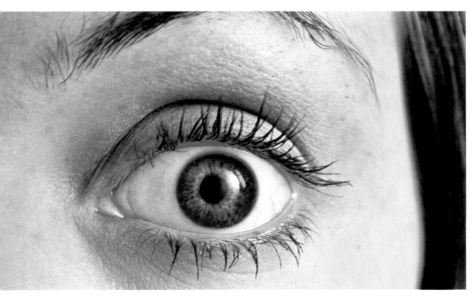

The outward signs of emotions affecting your body are familiar to everyone: the gasp of fright, the perspiration of anxiety, the widened eyes of surprise, and the common hot blush of embarrassment.

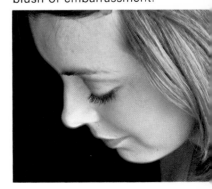

created by the brain. When you gasp in horror, or hold your breath in suspense; when your pupil enlarges in surprise; when you sweat from anxiety, or flush with embarrassment; when your heart pounds in fear, joy, or passion—these are all evidences of the mind/body link.

This link between mind and body operates through the *nervous system*. Scientists are still very far from understanding everything about the way this system works. We do know, however, that the part of the brain which we use for constructive thought is not all of the mind. While the *voluntary* part of our nervous system handles our conscious transactions with the outside world and the inner world of thought, the *autonomic* system works day and night to run the internal bodily functions that we do not need to think about. It controls heart beat, blood pressure, breathing, and the processes of digestion and elimination.

But in addition to maintaining a steady flow of essential services, the autonomic system also regulates these services to provide for sudden changes. In order to achieve this, the autonomic system works as two parts. The first of these parts is called the *sympathetic system:* it helps the body to go into action during emergencies. Supposing, for example, you find a hot pad, left on the stove, has caught fire. You must act at once to prevent a serious disaster. Many of your muscles need more energy in a hurry. The sympathetic system provides this extra energy by signaling the adrenal glands to give your body a strong shot of adrenalin. This increases the rate of breathing and heartbeat and shifts a large part of the blood supply to the muscles so that you can put out the fire.

Once the flames are safely out, and the danger is over, the other part of the autonomic nervous system—the *parasympathetic system*—helps restore your body to its normal state and prepares it for any further efforts that may be necessary. The parasympathetic system may therefore be thought of as working in opposition to the sympathetic

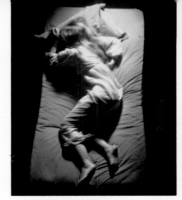
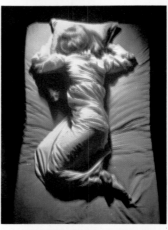
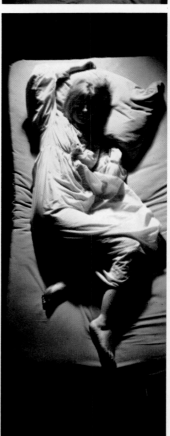
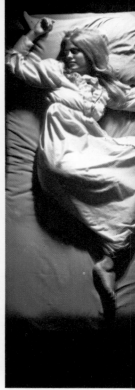
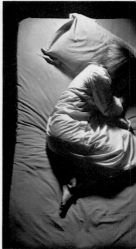
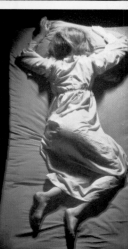

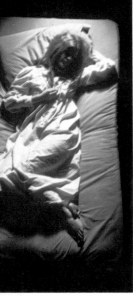
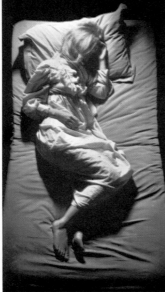

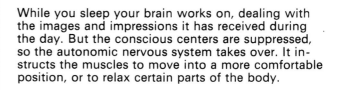

While you sleep your brain works on, dealing with the images and impressions it has received during the day. But the conscious centers are suppressed, so the autonomic nervous system takes over. It instructs the muscles to move into a more comfortable position, or to relax certain parts of the body.

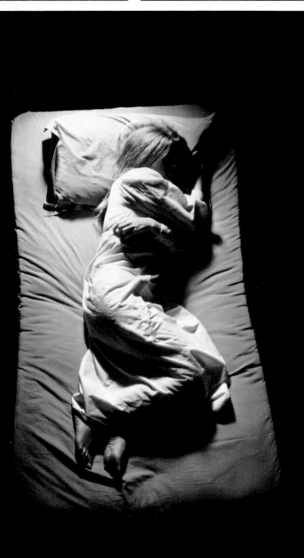

system, checking or counterbalancing it. It slows the heartbeat, makes breathing deeper and more regular, and starts up digestion that was temporarily halted during an emergency. The parasympathetic system also stimulates the mechanisms that control defecation and urination.

Ordinarily all this goes on without any conscious effort on our part, just as if the autonomic nervous system were quite separate from our consciousness. This seeming separation acts as a safety device built into our brains, for if the torrent of internal information necessary to keep our bodies working properly were to reach the conscious centers of the brain, we should all go crazy. Fortunately there is a barrier that holds back messages that are not important enough to engage our thought. The barrier also promotes sleep. When we are tired, it holds back impulses so that the conscious centers are not stimulated. The way is then clear for these centers to become inactive, and we fall asleep.

Near the brain barrier lies the *thalamus*. This is the location of sensations of pain and pleasure. Close to it is the *hypothalamus*—one of the main areas controlling the autonomic nervous system. Most of the time the hypothalamus acts without passing on information to the conscious areas of the brain. But as in all parts of the brain, impulses do not travel in one direction only. States of excitement, fear or anger in the conscious centers communicate themselves to the hypothalamus. This results in sweating, increased production of hormones, and changes of pulse rate and breathing.

Take as an example the stomach which

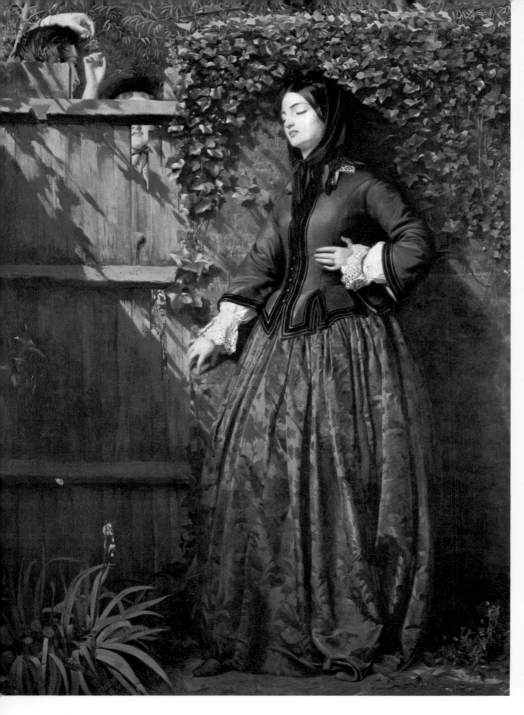

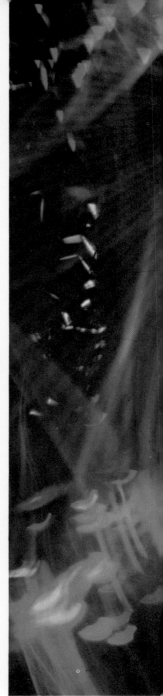

doctors call the number one target organ for emotional problems. You already know that strong emotions, worry, stress, and so forth, can have a powerful effect on the stomach. The familiar "butterflies in the stomach" that we so often feel in excitement is just one example. Now consider the situation in which a woman believes she is in great danger. The danger may be an actual physical threat to safety, or it may be a real or imagined danger to her inner self, such as a feeling of inadequacy, or the fear of losing her husband's love.

The idea that produces the sense of danger is a function of the voluntary nervous system. Her thinking brain, in turn, signals immediately to the hypothalamus which causes the adrenal glands to secrete hor-

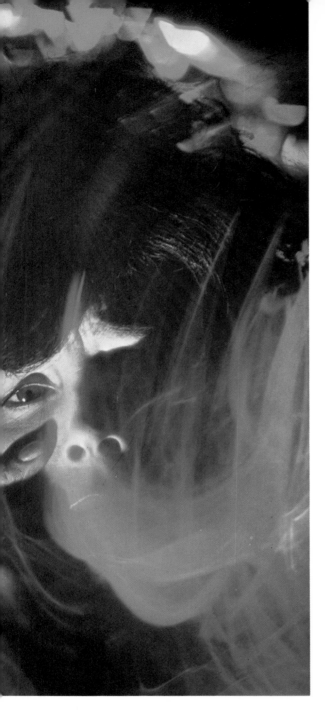

Far left; the physical pain brought on by love gone wrong is a common experience in life. It might be typical of the Victorians to depict a scene of heartbreak. But even today, a woman can suffer the cold misery caused by overhearing the man she loves declaring himself to someone else.

Left: most headaches are the result of simple nervous tension that pulls thousands of tiny muscles taut in your shoulders, neck, and jaw.

mones that prepare the body for fight or flight. The effects of these hormones are then felt by the autonomic system which brings about the changes in the body to prepare it for aggressive action.

But suppose our troubled woman can't find a way out of her frustration, or, like Shirley, for some reason doesn't dare let go and express her fears. Her body is con-tinuously under stimulation, ready for aggressive action, but her conscious mind tells her to repress any open expression of self-assertive hostile impulse. Such a prolonged interior battle without a means of release can upset many of her body functions.

Unrelieved threat, stress, or frustration can produce all kinds of digestive disorders, from nervous indigestion and diarrhea to stomach ulcers and colitis, all of which are becoming more and more common among women. Prolonged states of unexpressed and unrelieved aggression may also result in headaches and backaches, and even rheumatoid arthritis, all stemming from continuously tensed muscles. Emotional stress has also been known to interfere with the functions of the liver and kidneys, which can cause dangerous accumulations of poisonous substances in the body.

Sometimes anxiety and frustration, instead of producing any obvious bodily symptoms, result in an overwhelming feeling of fatigue. A woman who is worried, depressed—or even just plain bored—will probably not get sleep of the right quality to rest her conscious brain. She may suddenly feel as if she had barely enough energy to get around. There are no physical causes for this kind of fatigue. It has been created entirely in the brain.

So it is true. Your brain does have a great deal to do with your health, but knowing this, there is much we can do to keep body and mind working in harmony to produce a sense of genuine well-being. Let's now look at some of these positive ways in which we can make our mind our chief ally in promoting and maintaining good health.

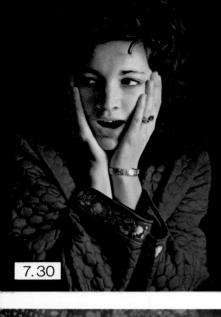

7.30

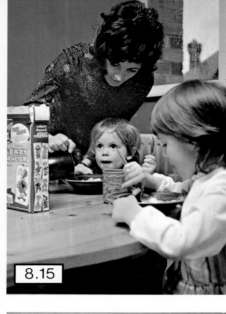

8.15

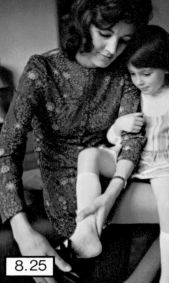

8.25

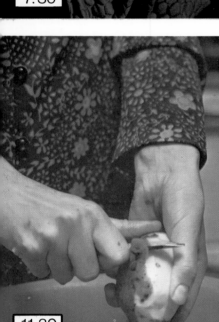

11.30

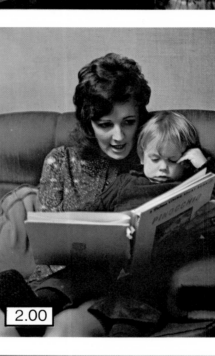

2.00

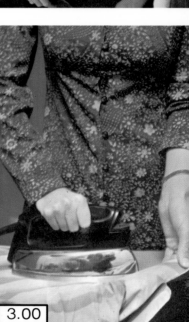

3.00

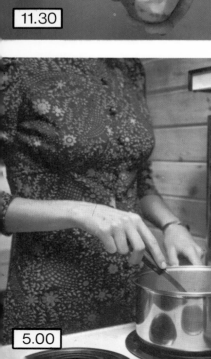

5.00

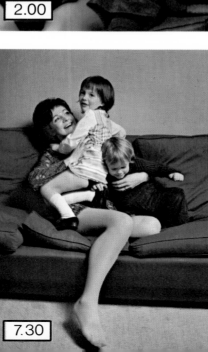

7.30

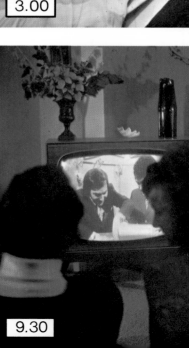

9.30

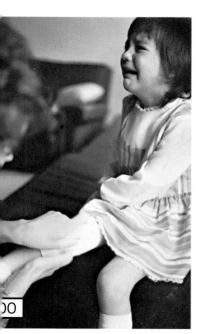

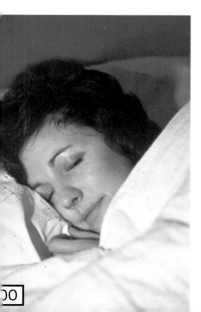

Think Well

3

Often for the housewife with young children each day seems an unchanging repetition of the day before. Meals have to be prepared, shopping done, and housework fitted in every day of the year. For most women there are times when even a wonderful family and a beautiful home do not seem to compensate for the never-ending round of jobs that have to be done again and again, day after day.

Nobody will argue with you if you say it's a tough world. It is. Life in this late 20th century is speeded up. The world is smaller. Problems can touch us from a great distance. We not only have to worry about what is going on at home, but also what is happening halfway around the world. Life in a complex modern society makes ever-increasing demands on our time, our energy, our attitudes and our emotions. Even the regular round of day-to-day living—earning enough money, coping with ever-rising prices, resolving the conflicting demands of job and family, or deciding how best to bring up our children—takes a lot more careful planning than it once did. And because the changes in our society and culture move ahead unevenly, rapidly in some areas and seemingly not at all in others, figuring out what a woman could or should do can become very confusing.

What it all adds up to is stress. Life is full of stress; it's an emotional pressure cooker. You can't escape it. Consider, for example, the woman who has finished her housework for the morning. Her dishes are done, the beds are made, and her children are at school. She looks around her home, and thinks "I shall have to go through exactly the same routine again tomorrow. Where's it getting me? Is this all there is to life?" Then there is the young-middle-aged mother whose children are nearly grown-up and no longer need her so much. She may see the future looming emptily ahead but worry that she will never find the self-confidence she needs to go out and work outside the home again. Another woman worries about whether she should have a baby or continue with the job she enjoys. Can she combine working with raising a child and still be "a proper mother?" What about the single woman who is made to feel that she's odd if she is not married by age 25? Or the woman who is confused by the current emphasis on sexual freedom? Convinced that she is missing out on the sexual revolution—or that her marriage is not providing the degree of sexual satisfaction that she has heard or read about—she finally goes out and has an affair. Then she walks around with her emotions in a turmoil, maybe feeling guilty and anxious, wondering whether it was such a good idea after all. We can all supply many such examples of emotional stress from the experience of our own daily lives.

Since you cannot escape stress, what can you do? The answer is blunt and uncompromising. Manage, or suffer the consequences. What happens to you in this stressful world depends entirely on you, on your determination to manage. This does not mean, however, that you have to do it all alone, without help. The stresses are there. You can eliminate some with positive action on your own. And when the problems are too tough, you can turn to professionals for help.

There is one thing, however, that you dare not overlook. The longer you go without recognizing stress and taking some steps to deal with it, the greater the danger that considerable damage may be done. For if stress and tension are allowed to build up without release, a woman can literally worry herself sick. Then the symptoms of psychosomatic illness set in.

Sometimes these symptoms are not clearly

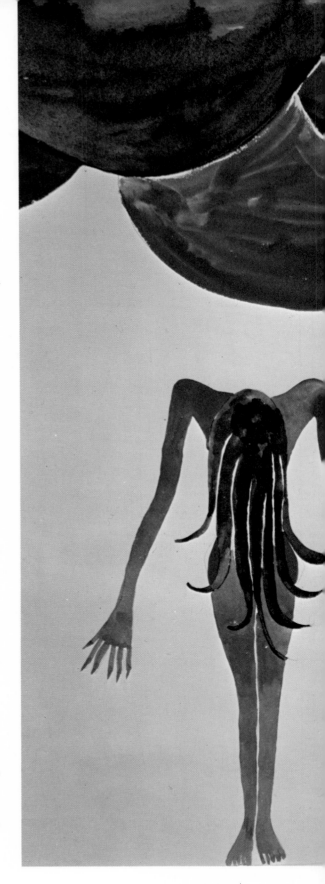

Left: in our society, the main responsibility for maintaining the home and family falls on women, who also increasingly have outside jobs. Some women find such a load too heavy to bear, and suffer breakdowns as a result. A middle-aged woman in a state of acute depression painted this picture showing a deep-rooted despair.

defined. Take the case of Marjorie, the young mother of two sons under five. She found herself becoming increasingly tired and less able to cope with her housework or her children. She would wake in the mornings with so little energy that she could hardly bear to face the day. She dragged herself around doing less and less housework, and sometimes did not even bother to dress her children until her husband came home in the evening. Then one day, she just gave up trying altogether. With a sense of panic, she realized that she no longer even wanted to get out of bed.

Marjorie's case is far from rare. Doctors call it the "Tired Suburban Housewife Syndrome," although you don't have to live in the suburbs; you don't have to be married; you don't even have to be a woman to have it. But as many as half of all women patients seen by doctors are, to some degree, victims of this syndrome. They may

Right: considering the pressure-cooker stress of today's life, it is a hopeful sign that treatment for mental illness is losing its stigma, and is being accepted as help for a type of sickness that could happen to anyone. These figures for a one-year period show the number of women admitted to state and county mental hospitals as first-time patients. It becomes clear that a woman's most difficult periods are the years of early adulthood, and the time during which she must deal with her children's adolescence.

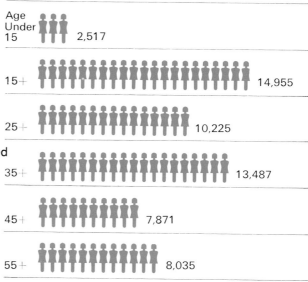

Age	
Under 15	2,517
15+	14,955
25+	10,225
35+	13,487
45+	7,871
55+	8,035

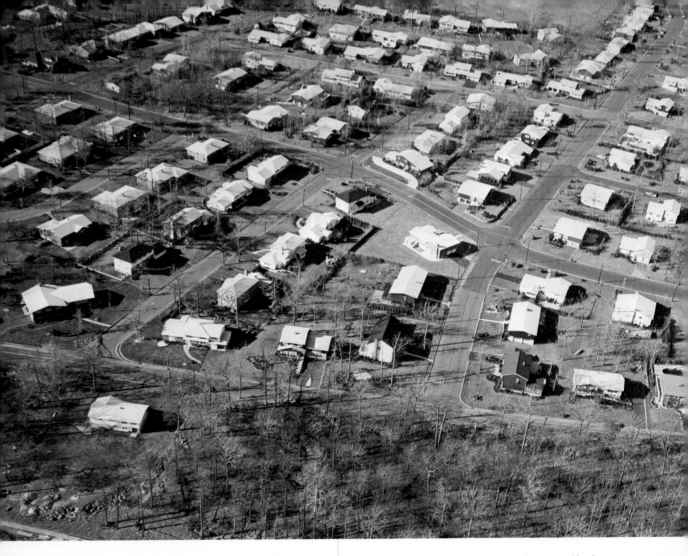

complain of tiredness, of inexplicable aches and pains, of a loss of sensation in parts of the body, or just vague and muddled feelings of misery and fatigue.

For the woman suffering from these complaints, medication may bring some temporary relief. But drugs do not attack the root cause of the trouble. For basically the problem is one of boredom: the boredom of being forced to follow the same routine day after day, year after year, without let-up, escape, variety or challenge. And boredom is stress. The only effective solution is to attack that stress directly. In extreme cases, naturally, psychiatric care is required. But very often a woman can, with determination, handle this stress fairly successfully in herself.

Let's now look at some of the suggestions doctors have made for coping with stress and see how they can best be applied to our own particular problems.

Know Yourself: The first step in living a truly healthy life is to accept yourself. Remember that the unconscious part of your brain knows exactly who you are. Every time you act in ways that conflict with your true self, the automatic nervous system will exact a toll.

The best way to find out who you are is to do some tough, honest self-analysis in which you put the proper names to things. If you feel that your family is taking you for granted, say so. If you feel that life is slipping you by, say that too. If you find your job or your homelife unbearably dull, admit it. The first step in relieving stress is to recognize that it exists. But don't just stop at saying that you feel put-upon, neglected, bored, or whatever.

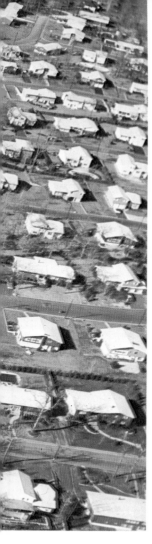

The streets of houses that are all variations on the same pattern are a familiar part of the ordinary suburban landscape: each house with its occupants living their everyday lives, often isolated by distance from the larger family unit that, in earlier days, would have given company and support.

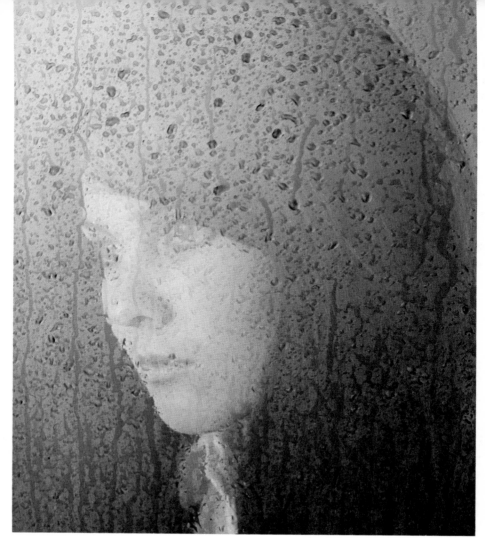

Try to discover just what is making you feel that way. Don't be surprised if the answers are slow in coming. Being honest with yourself—really letting your conscious mind hear what has been stored away for so long—takes time and practice.

Once you have recognized your problems, see what you can do to solve them by yourself. The solutions you choose will, of course, depend on your own individual case. But a few examples may help you to see how other women have worked their problems out.

Elsa complained that she simply had too much to do. Running her home was keeping her busy 18 hours a day. It was rare that she could ever manage to find a baby-sitter and go out with her husband to the movies, or a party. And when she did go to a party,

Many housewives of today feel trapped—as if the windows of their world look out only on their backyard fence. In a woman desperate with loneliness and boredom, emotional tension can build up to a point at which she gets physically ill in the same way that she might become sick from germs.

she found that she had nothing to talk about. Who would be interested in the fact that Junior had fallen over and cut his lip, that the serviceman hadn't turned up to fix the washing machine, that she had ironed half-a-dozen shirts, or found a new quick way of making Mexican rice?

She began to feel that she was turning into a drudge, wearing herself out day after day with nothing to show for it. But she was a methodical person. So she made a list of her week's activities, noting down which of them she disliked most and which she didn't really mind doing. And then she looked for ways of cutting down on the boring chores with a view to making time for her own interests.

She found, for example, that she loathed the never-ending round of shopping for food, cooking, and doing the dishes. So she tried shopping less often, and discussed with a neighbor the possibility of going into partnership to buy a freezer and sharing bulk-buying facilities. She and her neighbor managed to find two other housewives who wanted to join in the bulk-buying plan, and who also suggested setting up a baby-sitting exchange. Elsa also began cutting down on lengthy menus that kept her perspiring over the stove for hours. She also enlisted her eldest child's help in doing the dishes, setting the table, and straightening his own room.

At the end of it all, she found that she had saved a little time, but suddenly she didn't know what to do with it. Then one evening, looking through some old snapshots, she remembered that she had always enjoyed taking photographs. She got out her camera again and tried taking just a few pictures each day. Then she arranged for her husband to take care of the children for one night a week while she went to a class in photography. Gradually she began to find that she was building her daily schedule around her new interest, working out ideas as she went about her work, and getting through her routine faster because she had something to look forward to at the end of it.

Louise, too, was overworked—but for a different reason. Her children were all in their teens, but she still seemed to be doing as much for them as ever. It took Louise some time to realize why she was putting so much effort into running her home. The plain fact was that she was trying to make herself as indispensable as possible to her family because she dreaded the day when her children would no longer need her care and she would feel unneeded in her own home. She made up her mind that this was no good for her or her family, and that the answer might lie in seeking a job outside the home. But what could she do?

Before her marriage, she had worked in an office, but she didn't have any special skills. And the business world, she felt, had changed so much while she had been away from it, that she wondered if she would ever be able to cope. But she forced herself to go and take a course in typing, and later landed a part-time job. This was not the end of her troubles, however. She found office life dull and impersonal. "I need to be with people," she explained. And this thinking finally led her to apply for a job in a big local store. There she found the work tiring, but enjoyable because it brought her into contact with a wide variety of people and

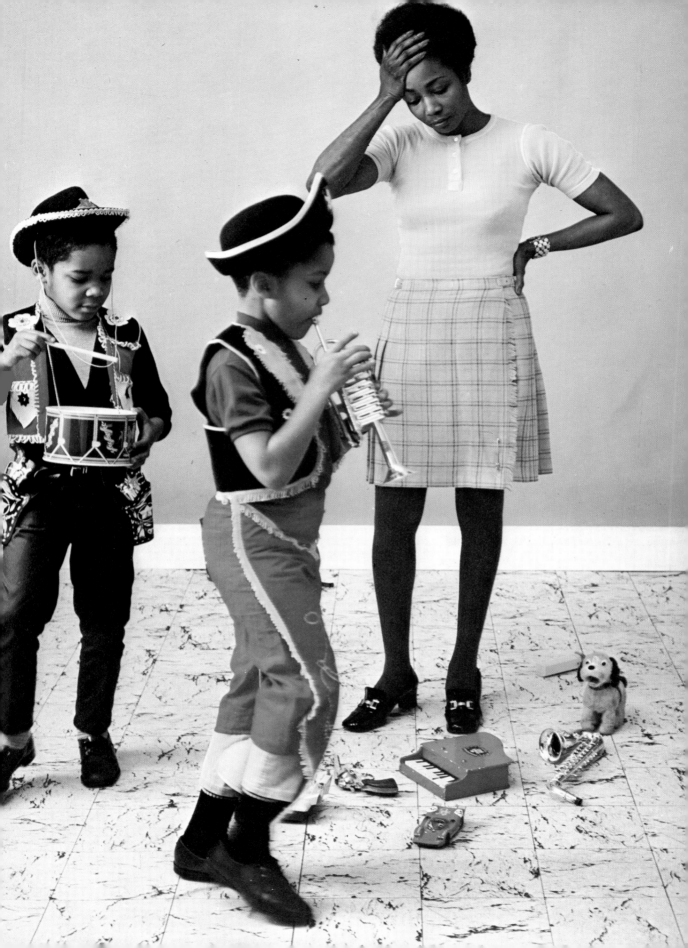

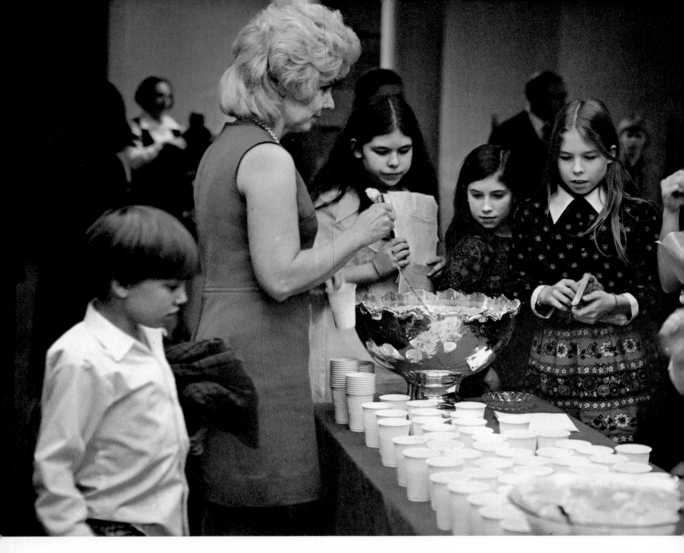

Above: volunteer work of some kind—such as helping at a school party—is a way in which many women keep contact with the outside world. Even during the years when a mother is most closely tied
to home, she can usually find a few free hours.

problems. "I'm so glad I took the plunge
and went out to work," she said. "Now, if
there's a family crisis going, at least I'm not
doing the dishes and thinking about it all
day. At work I have to deal with completely
different problems. And when I get home,
I may still act stupidly, but at least I have a
fresh outlook on things."

Learn to Escape: It is sometimes best to
handle problem situations by meeting them
head-on. Under some circumstances, there
may be nothing quite so good for the spirit as
unrelenting hard work. But most doctors
today believe that occasional side-stepping

of your problems and work is beneficial.
Many women set themselves too high a
standard, either at the office or in the home,
and find that they are regularly working
themselves to the point of exhaustion. At this
stage, family life suffers and emotions are set
on edge. So, although you want to do the
best job you can, try to organize your work
so that you can put some things off until
tomorrow—and gain time to devote to
yourself.

Every woman knows that there is no end
to the things that could be done in a house—
but there is an end to the things that should
be done to ensure a fair degree of comfort
and preserve your sanity at the same time.
Don't think that your family will suffer
from any short-cuts that you decide to take
in your daily routine, for the more contented

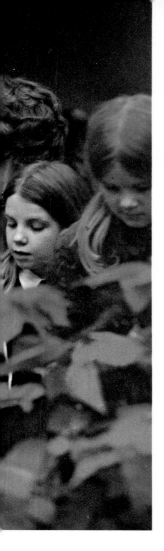
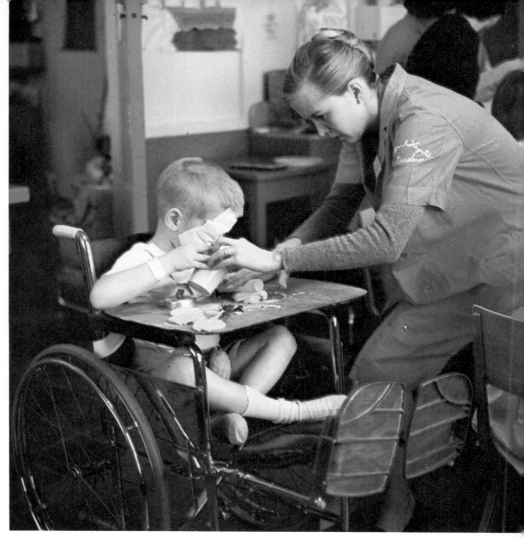

you are, the happier they will be.

If you grouse about the day's workload for the first hour or two after you get up, this automatically gears your mind to feelings of depression. So instead, try to cultivate positive thoughts of how to make your day brighter. Maybe you could arrange a lunch with a friend you haven't seen for years. Or plan a surprise for your husband or children. Or start a program of exercises to help you feel fitter and more relaxed.

Above all, introduce as much variety and interest as you can into your life. Plan your schedule to balance routine tasks that must be done with activities that you enjoy. Check over your interests and find ways of fitting them into your life. Is there some hobby that you used to like? Then take at least a small step toward doing it again.

Above: one of the tried and true ways of bypassing your own frustrations is to concentrate attention on someone else's problems. There are few things more rewarding than spending some time in amusing a hospitalized child. It will do both of you good.

Are you completely tied to the house? Then could you keep your hand in with the job you used to have by, say, practicing your typing once or twice a week? Or start planning what sort of work you might like to do when your children are grown-up, and read up on the sort of information you might need? Or can you, perhaps, find the time to contribute to a community activity, such as volunteer hospital work? If this idea attracts you, there are countless social service agencies near you that would value your contribution.

Bring your family in on the discussion and

53

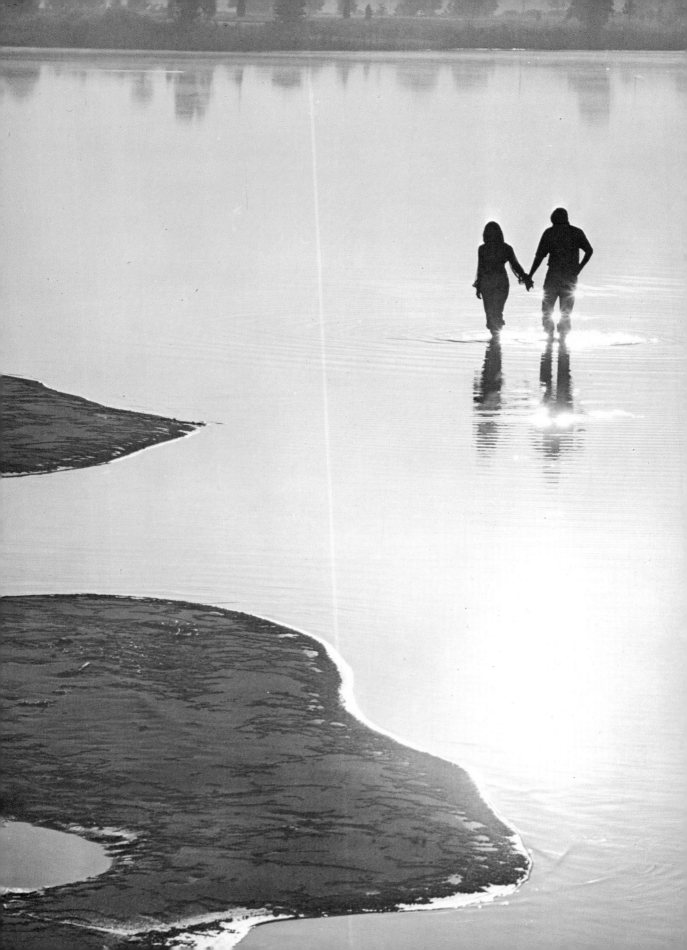

enlist their cooperation. Talk it over with other women, too. They have the same problems, whether they are full-time housewives or have a job outside the home as well.

Whatever you do, get away from it altogether once in a while. Can you manage to spend some time alone? A morning or afternoon walk is one good way of getting in touch with yourself, away from everybody, and exercise all at the same time. If possible, according to many health authorities, it is best for the whole family to take two shorter vacations than one longer one. And, they say, let weekends be real breaks from routine. But don't do the same thing every weekend!

Learn to Relax: "It is wonderful to see how the greatest stress can be endured if periods of relaxation are interspersed at enough intervals," says American doctor Sara M. Jordon. And even if you find it difficult to get away from your daily routine, you can help relieve tension by learning to relax.

Most of us find it pretty hard to relax. But one quick and effective way is to tense up your muscles as hard as you can, and then let them go slowly. Or try lying flat on your bed or the floor, with a pillow under your knees and head. Breathe quietly and regularly and let your muscles go limp as if your body were "melting" into the floor. Just 10 minutes of this relaxation can be wonderfully refreshing and also help you to get a good night's sleep.

British doctors have recently discovered that relaxation exercises designed for pregnant women are a tremendous help to patients suffering from migraine and other headaches caused by nervous tension. And

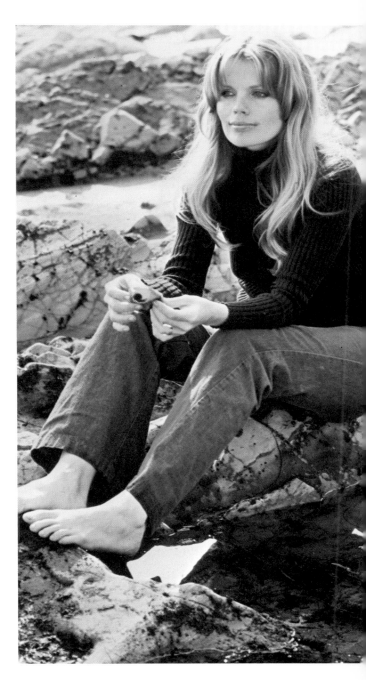

there are many other relaxing exercises you can try (see Chapter 6). Remember, too, that if you feel tired and irritable toward the end of the day, it is a good idea to change into loose comfortable clothes, or take a long, soothing bath to relax yourself before you go to bed.

Learn to Work Off Your Anger: Science tells us that every time you get angry your body reacts. Your sympathetic nervous system prepares you for aggression, or the parasympathetic system causes a kind of psychologic retreat. Either way, chemical balance is destroyed. If you are often angry and remain so, sulking and smoldering, you are getting yourself prepared for one or more mind-caused reactions.

If you feel yourself becoming angry and you tend to stay that way, Dr. Clement Martin recommends that you pitch into some physical activity, fast. Gardening, baking bread, cleaning out the house, or taking a long vigorous walk, can help clear your mind of hostilities before they take their toll. And don't save exercise for emergency purposes only, says Dr. Michael of the University of California, but do it as often as possible. Pick something that you really enjoy, like swimming or dancing—an activity that is strenuous but not tiring, and works your whole body. Other doctors recommend doing something with your hands, such as crafts, painting, or writing, which helps your brain switch from anger to a creative activity in which you can become really involved.

Learn to Express Your Feelings: Modern society being what it is, tends to value the even-tempered, compliant, predictable personality. And most of us are taught practically from birth to be ashamed of displaying our emotions. But the emotions are still there. And if there is any one cause of psychosomatic ills it is unexpressed, bottled-up emotion. Joy, passion, sorrow, fear, and anger all demand some kind of mind/body reaction. If we don't find a release for our emotions, the body suffers.

So learn how to let yourself go. Take anger,

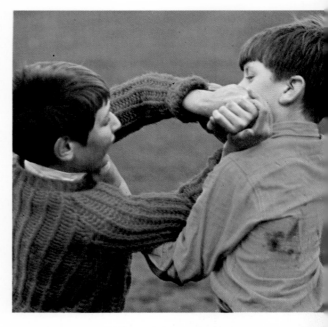

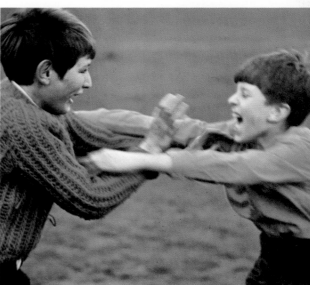

Some of us learn too well to suppress the wild free-for-all aggression that we see in children, and the resulting tension eats away inside us, often turning to bitterness. There are times in life when you should shout and be unashamedly angry.

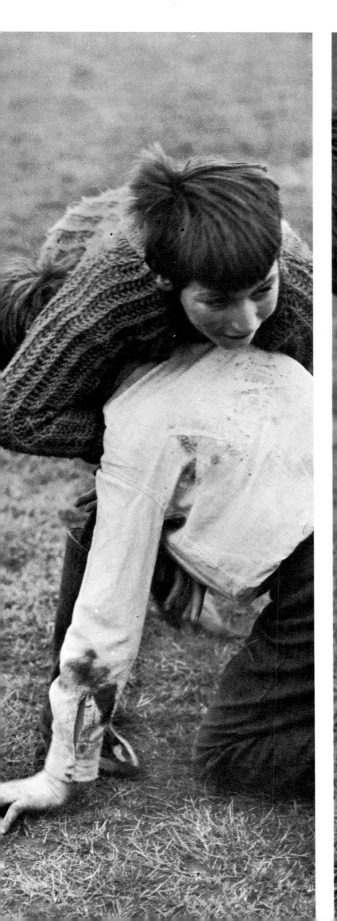
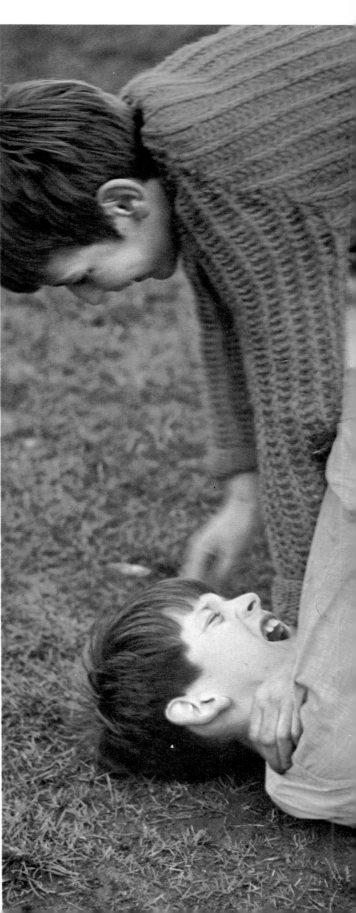

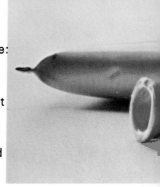

Some things don't change: the children squash the toothpaste in the middle, no matter what you say, and your husband will not pick up his clothes ever. You might as well accept these things. Pick up the clothes, fix the tube—and laugh if you can. Life will be happier that way.

for example. Some people find that a little shouting now and then will relieve their feelings like nothing else. But others quite naturally fear the effect of such flare-ups on good relationships. Perhaps one of the easiest ways to handle anger short of making a bitter scene, is to put into words how angry you feel and why. Suppose you were to tell a friend, "This is the UMPTEENTH TIME that my husband has fallen asleep in front of the TV and left me to do all the dishes and put the kids to bed. And I'm so furious that I simply have to tell someone about it before I burst!" That's more likely to do you good than having a bitter argument with your husband over it.

Sometimes, of course, the reasons for anger or other emotions are less straight-forward. They may even stem from un-resolved grievances that lie way back in the past. But once you have recognized that they exist, don't lock them away inside yourself. The safest way to ease your mind is always to talk your troubles over with some independent person whom you can trust.

Reorganize Your Life to Avoid Minor Irritations: Life is full of minor irritations, but no rule says you have to put up with all of them. Often it is a series of nagging little annoyances that keep us in a constant state of tension. Perhaps you are always mislaying things, forgetting what you went to the store for, missing the bus, paying your bills at the eleventh hour, or snapping back at the least provocation. Strangely enough, such irritations may be so much a part of our daily life that it seems hard to avoid them, and we suffer annoyance as if it were essential to

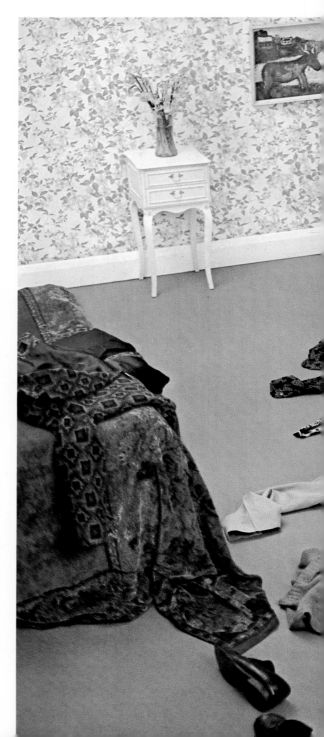

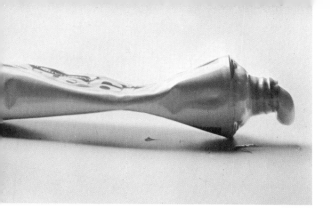

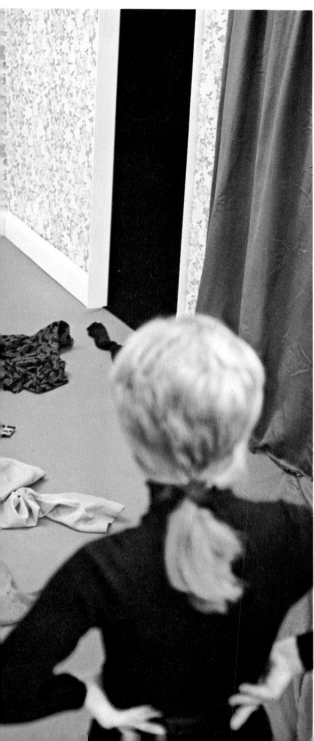

our life's routine. But if this is part of your life, ask yourself which is more important, your health or some effort to change things around? Try to take the long-term view and to insulate yourself against petty irritations by cultivating your sense of humor.

Learn to Accept the Other Person's Shortcomings: In short, learn to take some things as they are, because you may not be able to change them. Try to be tolerant and adopt a flexible attitude. The end result will be greater understanding. If, for example, you married a shy, quiet, home-loving man, it is no use blaming him for not being the life and soul of the party whose sparkling wit is the envy of your friends. This goes back once again to your own internal dialogue. The more you understand yourself, the less you will feel the need to change everybody else to meet your requirements.

Maybe you feel that none of this advice is any help. You feel your life is a tangle, and that things are getting worse instead of better. Then it's time to talk things over with someone who is a trained listener. If there are physical symptoms, the first place to go is to your doctor. Otherwise, a psychiatrist or other trained counselor is the person best qualified to help you work out a solution to your problems.

Remember, there is a way out. Despite all the stresses of this pressurized world, there is no need to make yourself sick through unpositive thinking. You *can* handle tension. And you can find a variety of ways to channel away the inevitable psychic tension that could otherwise hurt you. With or without outside help, you can think your way to a happier, healthier life.

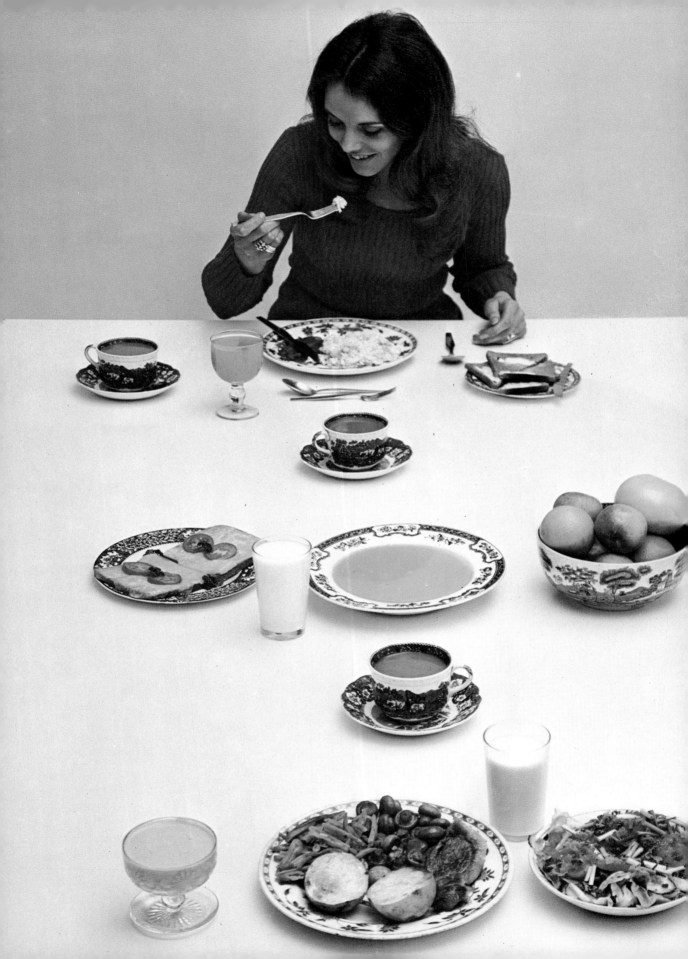

Eat Well
4

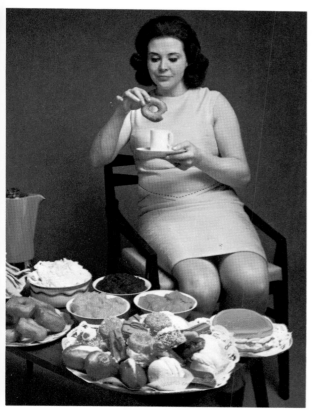

We seldom visualize all the food we eat during the course of a day as a total quantity, in one great heap. We tend to have a convenient amnesia to help us forget the bits and pieces that we tuck in between meals. But it is the whole pattern of your eating that makes up your diet, not the particular things you have for breakfast, lunch, and dinner. Left: these foods add up to about 2,100 calories, just right for a normally active woman's body. Above: junk foods do little to satisfy the nutritional needs of the body, and quickly add on fat.

Ann is a happily married woman with a weight problem. "My main trouble is that I can't bear to see food go to waste," she explains. A busy mother of three, Ann finds herself constantly finishing up her children's leftovers—a potato that isn't worth saving, a spoonful of ice cream, or a piece of apple pie. Ann feels that she spends most of her time cooking, since her children and her husband usually need their meals at different times. Often, she doesn't join them at the table but eats a few slices of toast for breakfast after the family has gone out, and finishes up whatever is left after her youngest child has been home from school for lunch. By mid-afternoon, she is usually tired and hungry and eats a snack with the children after school. She cooks a good filling meal for her husband in the evening, which she usually manages to share. At 33, Ann feels that she has lost her figure, and lately she has been making valiant efforts to diet. First of all, she cut out eating with her husband in the evening. But that didn't seem to help. So, in desperation, she tried almost starving herself altogether for a few days. Before the end of a week, however, she felt so worn out and miserable that she sat down and ate a whole box of candy. And the next day, she went back to her old eating habits.

Mary, on the other hand, never eats very much. In her late 50's, she was recently widowed and lives alone. Her son and daughter are married with families of their own and live too far away to visit her often. "Most of the time, I'm on my own," says Mary, "and I've just got out of the habit of cooking. After all, there's no pleasure in preparing food just for yourself." Usually,

Mary waits until she feels hungry and then boils herself a few potatoes or maybe makes a scrambled egg. Now and again, she might have a TV dinner. But a lot of the time, she just snacks on cookies and eats nothing else all day, with a few cups of coffee to keep her going.

Mary is considerably underweight. Ann is overweight. But both women are suffering from malnutrition. They are living on badly-balanced diets that are not giving them the nourishment essential to good health and well-being. And overeating or "wrong eating" contribute as much to malnutrition as eating too little.

A woman's nutrition, according to Adelle Davis (considered by many to be America's foremost nutritionist) can "determine how you look, act, and feel; whether you are grouchy or cheerful, homely or beautiful, physiologically and even psychologically young or old; whether you think clearly or are confused, enjoy your work or make it a drudgery."

If your body machine is to work at the peak of its potential, you must supply its simple needs: protein for growth and repair of your chemical self; vitamins and minerals to control and coordinate its intricate systems; carbohydrates and fats to keep the body warm and supply most of the energy for all the work it has to do.

The basis of any adequate diet is protein, found mainly in meat, fish, eggs, milk, cheese, and, to some extent, in wholegrain cereals, nuts, and dried beans and peas. Protein is the unique chemical of life. Your body is made of protein. And all the hormones in your body, including the

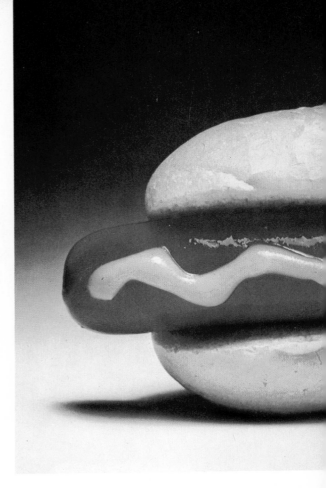

The traditional ballgame or after-movie snacks are no substitute for well-rounded meals. Your body must have many kinds of food to keep it healthy. Eating only one or two favorites that are tasty and quick to prepare can lead you into poor nutrition. Many of the snack type foods are also fattening.

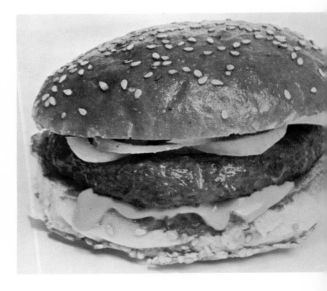

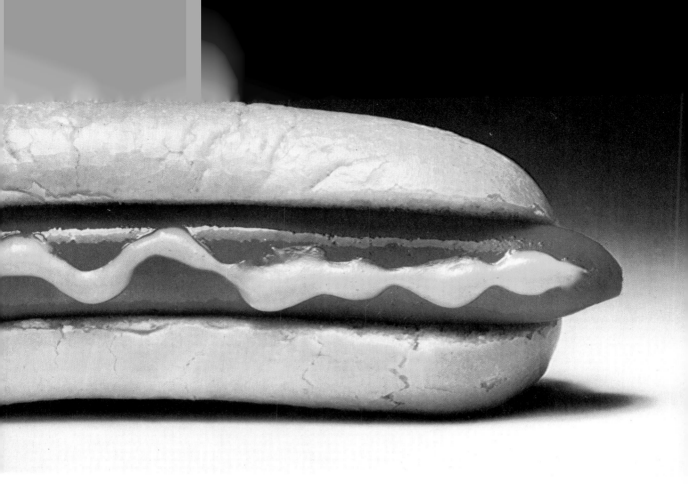

precious estrogens, are built on a protein base. Proteins also help to form the substances called *antibodies* to fight infection, and the chemicals known as *enzymes* which play an important part in digestion.

While we all need plenty of protein in our diet, we need only very small amounts of vitamins to preserve health and well-being. But these small amounts are vital. Without them, we could not survive for more than a few months at the most. For vitamins act as delicate balancing agents in our body cells and are essential to almost all body reactions. They also help to protect the body against disease and to build up health after an illness.

Vitamins are present in most of the food we eat, and, provided your diet is properly balanced, you should get all the vitamins you need. But vitamins can be destroyed in cooking, and you should keep a lookout for any possible deficiency. About 12 of the 40

or more vitamins so far discovered, are known to be essential to life. Five of these vitamins and some foods which contain them are listed in the chart on page 68. Experts have calculated our approximate needs for most of these vitamins and the chart on page 66 gives the *minimum* daily requirements of five of these for women of various ages.

Minerals are also essential to the body for building new cells and for controlling the chemical reactions that take place within them. They are particularly important for healthy bones, teeth, blood, skin, hair and nails.

Most minerals are needed in such tiny quantities that no diet would normally be deficient in them. There are, however, four important minerals of which you could just possibly run short. These are: sodium (found in salt), calcium (from milk and cheese), iron (from meat and eggs), and iodine (from fish and other sea foods and iodized salt).

Iron is particularly important for women because it helps make red blood cells and, since women regularly lose a certain amount of blood during their monthly periods, they need to take in more iron than men. Iron deficiency can also cause anemia, which because of the menstrual blood loss and the demands of pregnancy, is far commoner in women than in men. Most women can probably get enough iodine from sea food—either fresh, frozen or canned—but it is a good idea to make sure of an adequate supply by always using iodized salt.

Of all the food we eat, the largest constituent is water. A quart of milk, for example, contains over 87 per cent water, and an apple 84 per cent. Even a slice of bread is 35 per cent water. Few of the essential chemical reactions of life can occur without water, and water is also the cleansing medium that relieves your body of poisonous wastes. More than six pints of this water is lost each day as sweat and in urine. But this is easily replaced by water in food and the liquids that we drink. All healthy people have a very efficient mechanism for insuring that the body retains exactly the amount of water it needs. If you take in too much water, the exact amount of excess is excreted; if you take too little, you will feel thirsty and take in some more.

The next essential is a source of energy. Moving the body around requires a great deal of energy. So, too, do the internal movements of the intestines and heart; even thinking, feeling, and reacting consume some energy.

With the exception of vitamins, minerals and water, all foods contain energy. But, by far the greatest energy-suppliers are fats and carbohydrates. Foods containing sugar and starch, such as bread, potatoes, cakes, and candies are rich in carbohydrates. They give the body energy by being turned into glucose in the digestive tract. Some of this glucose is sent to the body tissues for immediate use. So, when we eat a piece of bread, the energy this provides is made available almost right away. Part of your

meal may thus provide you with the energy to digest the rest. After a meal, however, any glucose not needed for energy is stored in the liver. And when the liver is full, glucose is carried to other parts of the body and deposited as fat.

Fats are made from the same chemical units as sugars and starches, but they supply more than twice as much energy as the same weight of carbohydrates. They also provide some vitamins and play an important part in the working of body cells. Fats are found mainly in butter, lard, margarine, oils, and fried food, fat meat, some fish, milk, cream, cheese, chocolate, and ice cream.

Although an excessive amount of fat in a diet is also stored in the body as fat, the right intake of fat can provide some unexpected bonuses. Adelle Davis reports, for example, that when just two tablespoons of salad oil were added to the seemingly adequate diets of some women, they experienced increased sex interest, a decrease in menstrual problems and, in some cases, longed-for pregnancies.

Our bodies need all the nutrients that food provides, but they need them combined together in the right proportions. The key to healthy eating is balance. What then, is a well-balanced diet? The answer depends on numerous factors. A woman must keep in mind that her requirements will change with the level of her physical activity, her degree of health, age, weight, and, of course, if she becomes pregnant. She should know, for example, that her maximum vitamin requirement occurs during her childhood and teens, and during pregnancy. She hits maximum peak energy demand probably around the age of 15 and it begins to fall off sharply in her very early 20's. Her highest iron demand occurs between the ages of 13 and 20 and then drops off, so that she can usually obtain enough iron from her normal

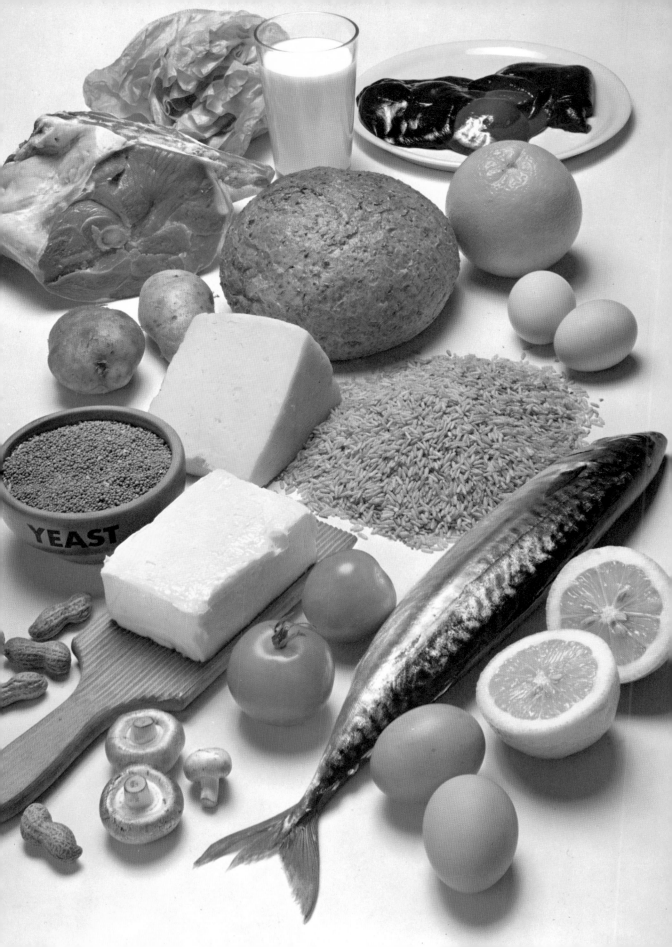

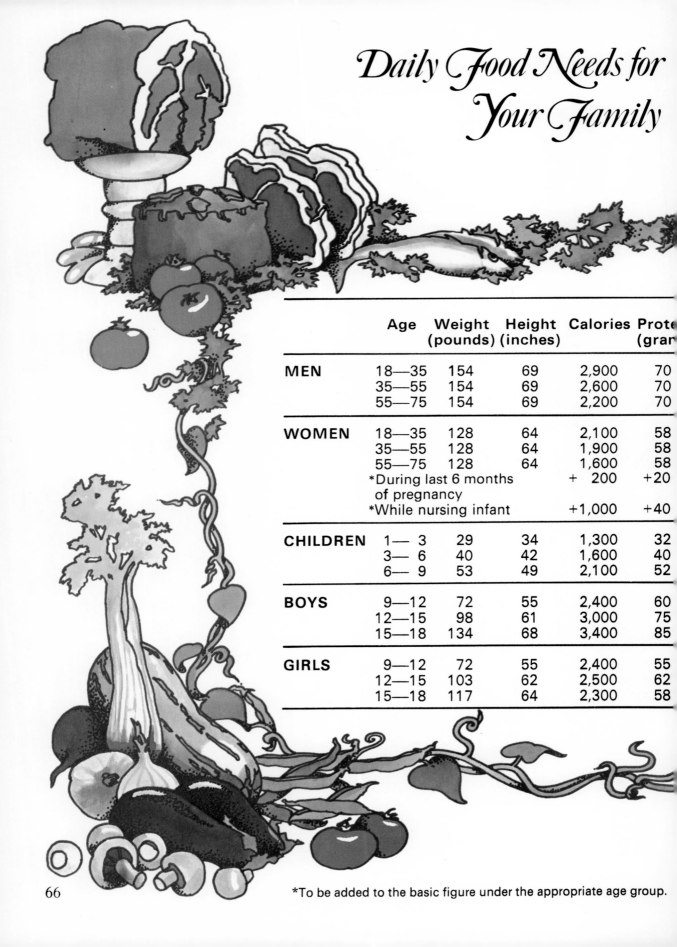

Daily Food Needs for Your Family

	Age	Weight (pounds)	Height (inches)	Calories	Prote (gran
MEN	18—35	154	69	2,900	70
	35—55	154	69	2,600	70
	55—75	154	69	2,200	70
WOMEN	18—35	128	64	2,100	58
	35—55	128	64	1,900	58
	55—75	128	64	1,600	58
	*During last 6 months of pregnancy			+ 200	+20
	*While nursing infant			+1,000	+40
CHILDREN	1— 3	29	34	1,300	32
	3— 6	40	42	1,600	40
	6— 9	53	49	2,100	52
BOYS	9—12	72	55	2,400	60
	12—15	98	61	3,000	75
	15—18	134	68	3,400	85
GIRLS	9—12	72	55	2,400	55
	12—15	103	62	2,500	62
	15—18	117	64	2,300	58

*To be added to the basic figure under the appropriate age group.

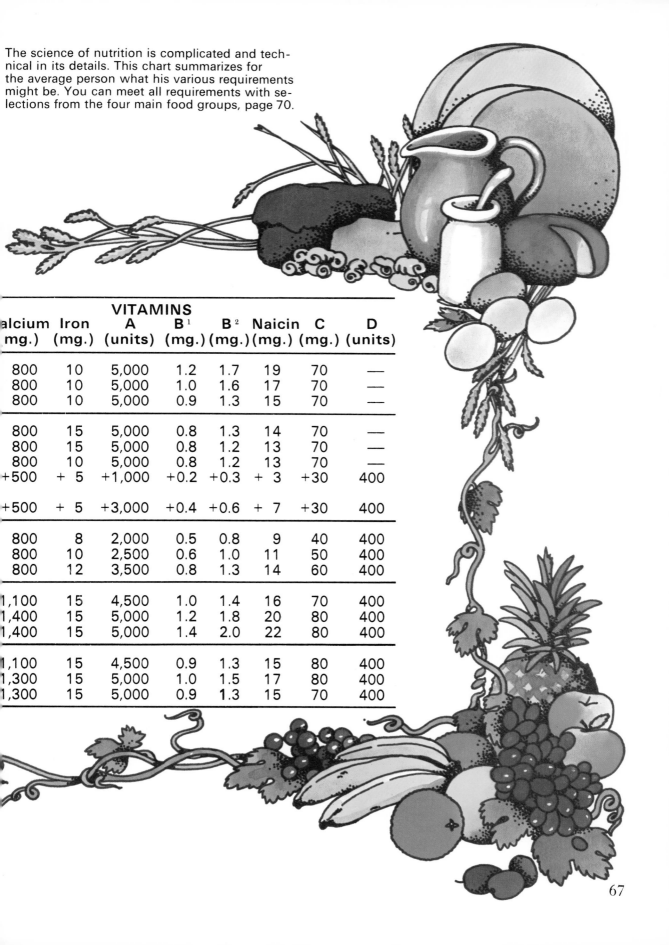

The science of nutrition is complicated and technical in its details. This chart summarizes for the average person what his various requirements might be. You can meet all requirements with selections from the four main food groups, page 70.

Calcium (mg.)	Iron (mg.)	VITAMINS A (units)	B¹ (mg.)	B² (mg.)	Naicin (mg.)	C (mg.)	D (units)
800	10	5,000	1.2	1.7	19	70	—
800	10	5,000	1.0	1.6	17	70	—
800	10	5,000	0.9	1.3	15	70	—
800	15	5,000	0.8	1.3	14	70	—
800	15	5,000	0.8	1.2	13	70	—
800	10	5,000	0.8	1.2	13	70	—
+500	+ 5	+1,000	+0.2	+0.3	+ 3	+30	400
+500	+ 5	+3,000	+0.4	+0.6	+ 7	+30	400
800	8	2,000	0.5	0.8	9	40	400
800	10	2,500	0.6	1.0	11	50	400
800	12	3,500	0.8	1.3	14	60	400
1,100	15	4,500	1.0	1.4	16	70	400
1,400	15	5,000	1.2	1.8	20	80	400
1,400	15	5,000	1.4	2.0	22	80	400
1,100	15	4,500	0.9	1.3	15	80	400
1,300	15	5,000	1.0	1.5	17	80	400
1,300	15	5,000	0.9	1.3	15	70	400

Those Vital Vitamins

This chart compares the vitamin content of one food with another, showing how much you would have to eat of each if you wanted to meet the daily requirement from one food alone. A study of it might help you fix in mind—and so shop for—the fruits, vegetables, and meats that are richest in vitamins.

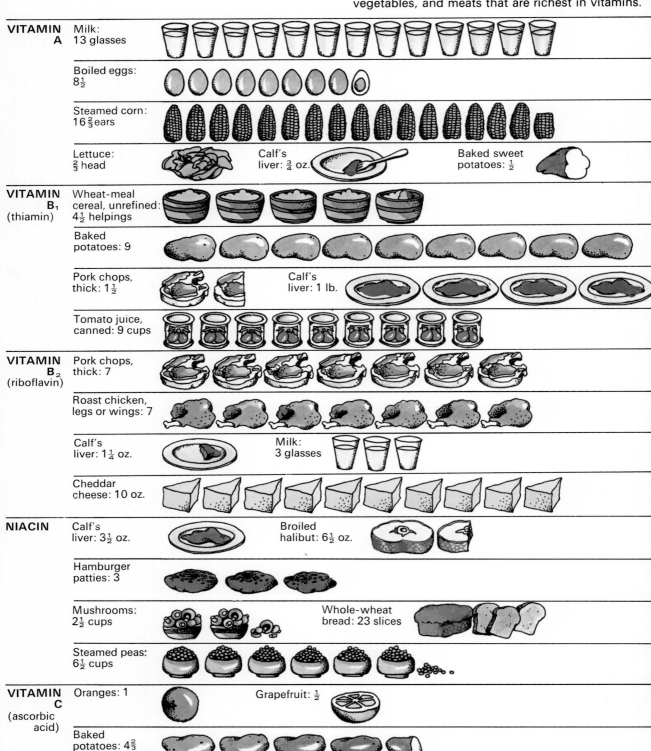

VITAMIN A	Milk: 13 glasses
	Boiled eggs: 8½
	Steamed corn: 16⅔ ears
	Lettuce: ⅔ head — Calf's liver: ¾ oz. — Baked sweet potatoes: ½

VITAMIN B₁ (thiamin)	Wheat-meal cereal, unrefined: 4½ helpings
	Baked potatoes: 9
	Pork chops, thick: 1½ — Calf's liver: 1 lb.
	Tomato juice, canned: 9 cups

VITAMIN B₂ (riboflavin)	Pork chops, thick: 7
	Roast chicken, legs or wings: 7
	Calf's liver: 1¼ oz. — Milk: 3 glasses
	Cheddar cheese: 10 oz.

NIACIN	Calf's liver: 3½ oz. — Broiled halibut: 6½ oz.
	Hamburger patties: 3
	Mushrooms: 2½ cups — Whole-wheat bread: 23 slices
	Steamed peas: 6½ cups

VITAMIN C (ascorbic acid)	Oranges: 1 — Grapefruit: ½
	Baked potatoes: 4⅔
	Raw tomatoes: 2 — Steamed cauliflower: 1

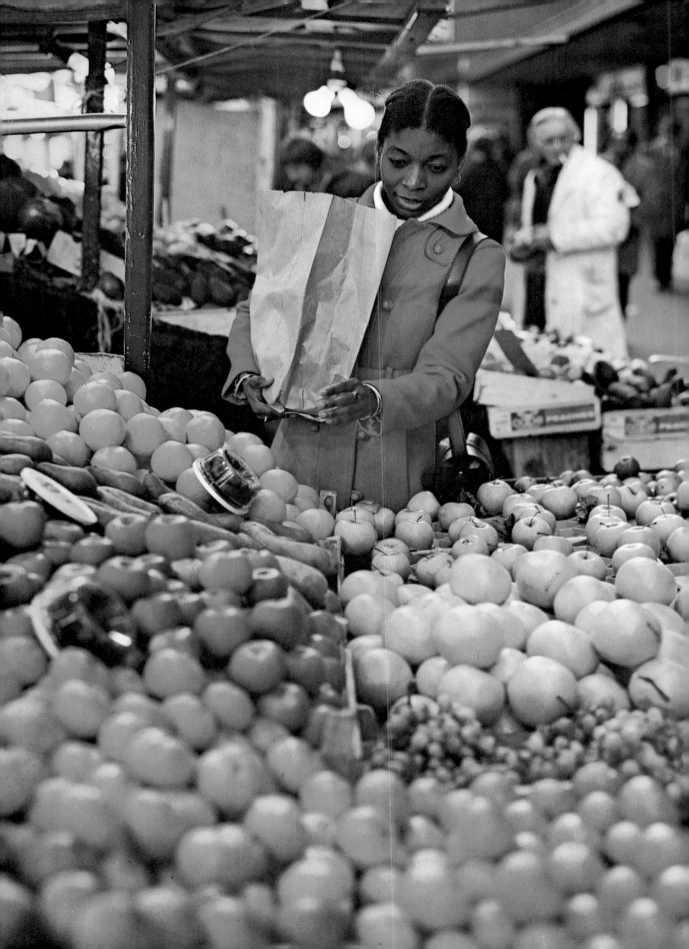

What's in Your Food

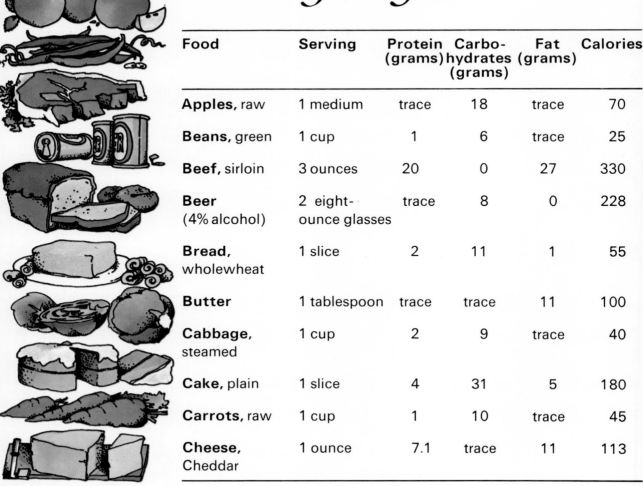

Food	Serving	Protein (grams)	Carbo-hydrates (grams)	Fat (grams)	Calories
Apples, raw	1 medium	trace	18	trace	70
Beans, green	1 cup	1	6	trace	25
Beef, sirloin	3 ounces	20	0	27	330
Beer (4% alcohol)	2 eight-ounce glasses	trace	8	0	228
Bread, wholewheat	1 slice	2	11	1	55
Butter	1 tablespoon	trace	trace	11	100
Cabbage, steamed	1 cup	2	9	trace	40
Cake, plain	1 slice	4	31	5	180
Carrots, raw	1 cup	1	10	trace	45
Cheese, Cheddar	1 ounce	7.1	trace	11	113

diet and will probably only need an iron supplement if she becomes pregnant. But her highest nutritional demands occur if she breast feeds after the baby is born. The table on page 66 shows the *minimum* recommended daily allowances of the chief food elements for men, women, and children at different stages of their lives.

But how can you be sure that you are getting all these essential elements in the right amounts each day? Fortunately, most of the foods we eat contain several of the essential nutrients. But we can make certain that we do not go short of anything by choosing our meals from four main groups established by nutrition experts. These four important groups are:

Group 1: Milk and cheese
(providing protein, many vitamins, and some minerals, especially calcium)
Group 2: Meat, fish, and eggs
(providing protein, some B-group vitamins and some minerals, especially iron and phosphorus)
Group 3: Vegetables and fruits
(providing vitamins, especially C and A, and, in many cases, iron and calcium)
Group 4: Butter and margarine
(providing Vitamins A and D)
Nutritionists suggest that you should have two reasonable helpings twice a day from

Proper nutrition is not just a matter of vitamins, because a good diet must also include protein, fat, and even that tricky carbohydrate. Your body must have all of these, and in the right amounts of each.

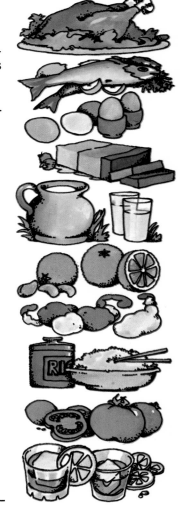

Food	Serving	Protein (grams)	Carbo- hydrates (grams)	Fat (grams)	Calories
Chicken, fried leg	3 ounces	25	0	15	245
Cod, broiled	3½ ounces	28	0	5	170
Eggs, boiled	2	12	trace	12	150
Ice cream	½ pint	6	29	18	300
Milk, whole	1 quart	32	48	40	660
Oranges, fresh	1 medium	2	16	trace	60
Potatoes, baked	1 medium	2	22	trace	100
Rice, white	1 cup	14	150	trace	692
Tomatoes, raw	1 medium	1	6	trace	30
Whiskey (86% proof)	1 ounce	0	trace	0	70

each of these groups. But if you eat enough milk or cheese, or both, you don't necessarily need any food from the meat group. As a general rule, they recommend that adults should drink 2 cups of milk a day and children 3-4 cups. All these foods should be eaten as nearly as possible in their natural state and should never be overcooked. Fresh food should always be chosen in preference to frozen or canned.

Once you have a good basis for your diet from all four groups, you can fill up with any other food you like—depending on how hungry you are and how slim you want to be. Foods like potatoes, pasta, bread and cereals (which should be made of whole-grain or enriched flour) will give you a few

more nutrients as well as energy. One exception, however, is sugar. It supplies energy, but it has no protein, vitamins or minerals to offer, and when it is not used for energy, it is laid down as fat.

Ideally the food you eat should provide your body with the exact amount of energy that it needs for its various activities. In order to plan an adequately balanced diet, therefore, we have to rate foods in terms of the amount of energy they release inside the body. As every woman knows, this energy is expressed in units called calories (short for Kilocalories), and a special calory count is given for every item of food.

Calories of food equal calories of energy. An average woman—a housewife, say—

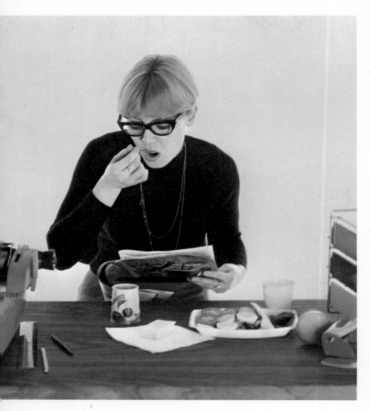

doing an average amount of work uses up about 2,000 calories a day. A man working in an office might need a few more calories— about 2,600. And a man with a more active job would probably use up as many as 3,500 calories.

Some people may take in as many as 2,500 calories in a single meal. And frequent snacks of cakes and candies can bring the daily total as high as 4,000 calories. But don't forget that if you eat more food than you use up, the excess will become fat. On the other hand, if you eat less food than you need, your body will draw extra energy from the fat deposits in your tissues—and you will lose weight.

This all adds up to the sad fact that we get fat for one reason only: because we eat too much. And overeating doesn't necessarily mean consuming vast quantities of food, but simply eating too much for our needs. All those excuses we like to make to ourselves—such as being born fat, having big bones, "gland trouble," or fluid retention— are, alas, unlikely to be at the root of our weight problems. You may have inherited a big frame, but it is up to you whether you put too much fat on it. As for glandular disturbances, these affect only a tiny minority of people, and usually produce many other uncomfortable symptoms apart from fatness. Similarly, fluid retention occurs only in people who have kidney disorders and, temporarily, in women during the premenstrual period. As we have seen, the body is well-equipped to keep a precise balance of fluid for its needs. This balance is, of course, often disturbed during the premenstrual phase, but the body rids itself naturally of such temporary excess fluid in the first few days of the menstrual cycle.

When exactly do extra pounds add up to overweight? Doctors define overweight as 20 pounds above the average weight for height and age. Thirty pounds over the average is called obesity. But most doctors agree that even 10 pounds above the average is dangerous to health.

Just as a guide, doctors say that you should be able to keep the figure you had when you were 20. That sounds pretty hard. But if you were fairly slim in your twenties and now weigh well over 10 pounds more than that, you can be pretty sure that you are overweight.

Overweight and obesity are now the commonest health problems in the Western world. Scientists estimate that 30 per cent of all Americans and 20 per cent of Europeans are obese (30 pounds above average weight). And, although overweight affects both sexes, it is more frequently found among women.

Why, then, do some women eat too much and become overweight? No one knows all

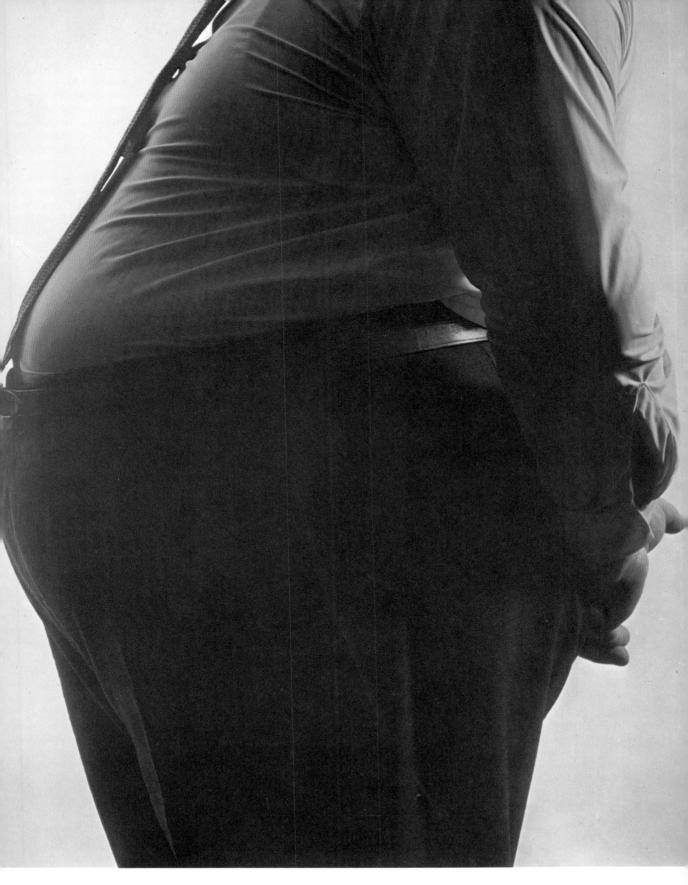

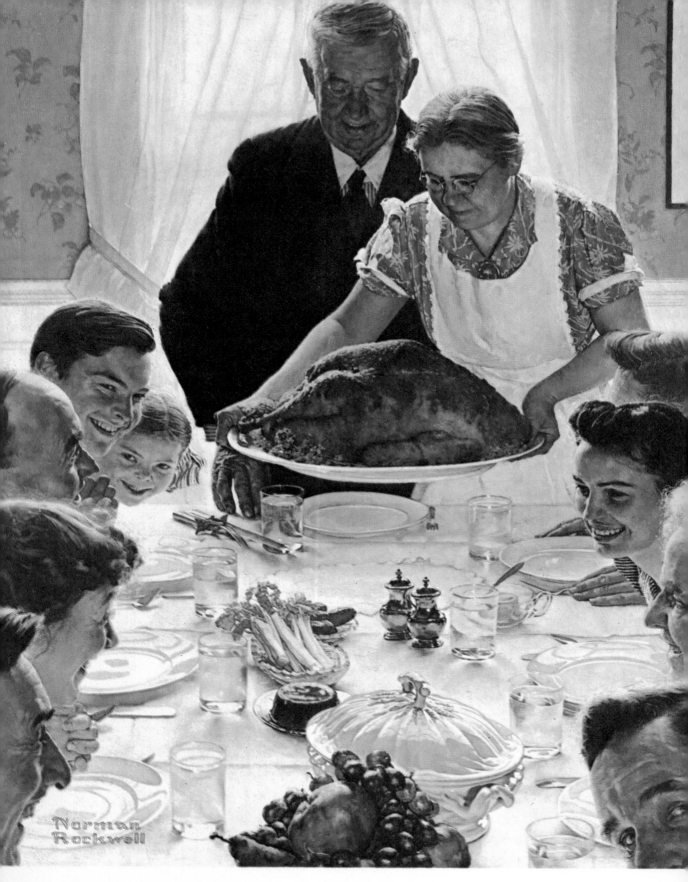

the reasons, but the experts agree that psychological factors are usually involved. Normally, the amount of food we eat is carefully controlled by a special "appetite center" in the brain which nutritionists call the *appestat*. The appestat makes sure that we eat just the right amount to give us the energy we need. But the appestat can easily be upset by emotional stress and by bad eating habits. And it will work less accurately if we do very little physical exercise.

Eating, as we all know, is far more than just a means of nourishing the body. For most of us it is a pleasurable experience. And it is an integral part of family and social life. When friends come to visit, we automatically offer them food and drink. Many social functions are centered around dinner—and it is usually a special dinner for the occasion.

In addition, most of us now do far less physical work, and ride rather than walk. Our leisure time has become far more passive, and is often interspersed with unnecessary snacks. Add to this the fact that we are constantly besieged by advertisements to nibble this, or eat that, and it is hardly surprising that so many of us are a good deal plumper than we should be.

Some people react to overwork and worry by overeating. For others, eating may be a form of addiction. And the foods to which they become addicted are usually the sweet and starchy fat-makers. Overweight or not, most of us tend to eat cakes, candies, ice cream, or chocolate because they taste good, rather than because we are hungry. And once we acquire a fondness for such foods, we find it desperately hard to change our eating habits.

Eating habits are usually formed in childhood. And some people overeat all their lives because that is what they were taught to do as children. Well-meaning or over-anxious mothers may overfeed their children in the mistaken belief that it is good for them, or even that plumpness is a sign of good health. Children are quick to see that one of the surest ways to make mother anxious is to refuse to eat, so that food may become a central issue in family rows and scenes. On the other hand, food is sometimes withheld from a child as a punishment. In this way, a child may identify food with love and security. And, later in life, eating may become a substitute for love, providing a source of comfort against disappointment, frustration, or unhappiness.

Once overeating has become a firmly entrenched habit, some people may use the resulting excess weight as an excuse to avoid unwanted contacts or activities. It is easy enough to fall into the vicious circle of eating because you are unhappy, bored, or lonely, and putting on weight to the point where you also feel physically unattractive, and so hide away from society, maybe filling the emptiness by eating some more.

Whatever the reasons for a woman becoming overweight, it is always possible and essential for her to return to more normal weight. The first step in this process, of course, is for her to recognize that she is overweight—a far more difficult process than you might think. Recent discoveries indicate that most people have something called a "body image"—a mental image of what their bodies look like which does not necessarily conform to reality. Many over-

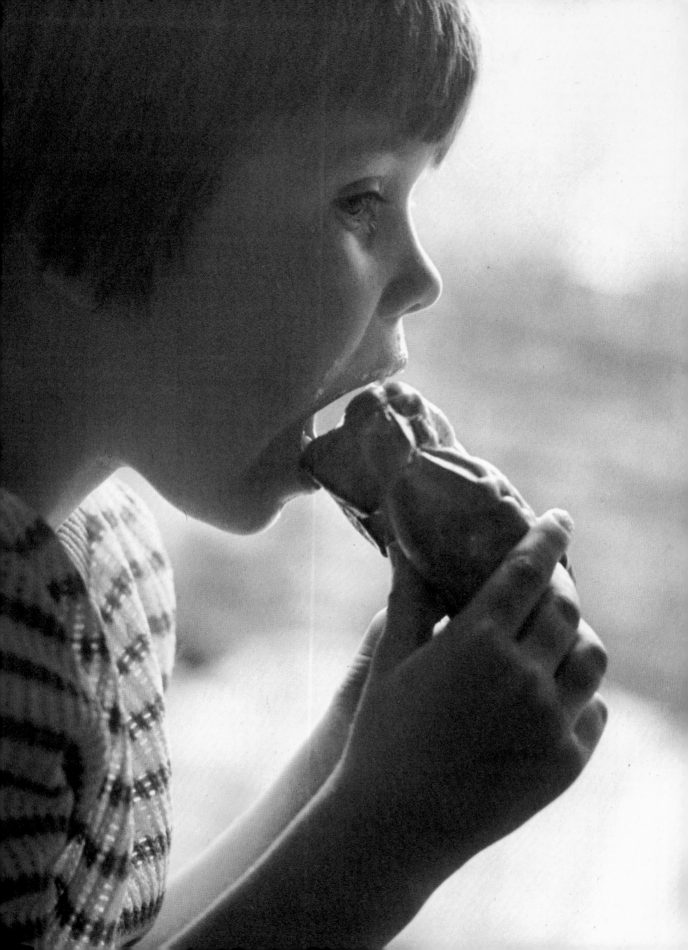

We carry through life the attitudes we learned about food as children. A piece of cake often stood for a good behavior reward. Often, too, our books showed animals enjoying splendid food at parties.

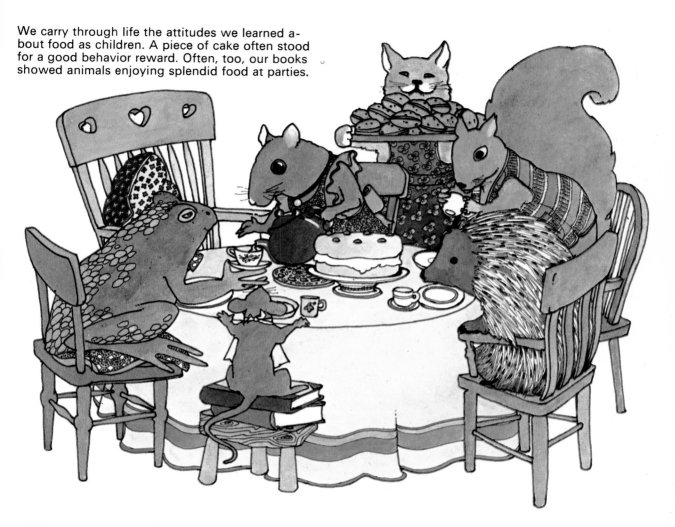

weight women continue to retain a body image of themselves formed when they were slim. They still think of themselves as being slim.

Once a woman sees for herself that she is overweight, and has undergone a thorough physical examination, her doctor will take a detailed history and then prescribe an appropriate reducing diet. In most cases, this involves not only the construction of a diet, and possibly the prescription of vitamin supplements and other medications, but also at least some mental reconditioning. Without all these elements, the cure will not work.

Unless there is some other complicating condition that absolutely requires immediate rapid weight reduction, the doctor will not prescribe a crash diet. Such diets require superhuman efforts to succeed and rarely have been known to work in the long run.

A woman should, in fact, be very wary of the many highly publicized crash diets, particularly those which emphasize the eating of only one food. As one doctor puts it, "If you eat one food, any food, you will lose weight. You will also get sick!" And there is a very real danger that the devotee of crash diets may starve her body of essential nutrients, thus disturbing her entire chemical balance.

A diet should not be for a short time. It must be forever. The ideal procedure, therefore, is to retrain the appetite to a new and permanent way of proper eating. This doesn't just mean eating less but also eating the right kinds of food. Then a weight balance will be achieved, giving all the right bonuses in terms of health and beauty.

For the woman who really wants to lose weight, the first step is to locate the eating habits that are causing most of the trouble—nibbling chocolate or candies during the day, having extra toast for breakfast, a drink after work, a snack while watching TV, or just a compulsion to finish up leftovers. Then she needs to choose a diet which is as close as possible to her old way of eating, so that she can get herself into new eating habits without feeling constantly hungry and miserable.

Since the basis of all weight reduction or weight maintenance diets is cutting down on the number of calories a person eats, the new food habits must place a far greater emphasis on the eating of proteins and a reduction in the intake of calorie-rich carbohydrates and fats.

Fat contains, weight for weight, twice as many calories as carbohydrate. And so many diets recommend cutting down severely on fat—eating no butter, fried foods, or salad dressing, for example. However, although this is an effective way of losing weight, many nutritionists agree that it is not the best way for everyone. Many people find a low-fat diet rather unpalatable and difficult to stick to. In addition, a lack of fat may make some people irritable and tired, reduce their powers of concentration, and cause skin problems. Some women do find that they do well with a low-fat diet, but since certain vitamins important to a woman's well-being are frequently derived from fats, vitamin supplements may be necessary during such a diet.

For most people a low-carbohydrate diet is usually more acceptable. And, as many carbohydrate-rich foods also contain fat, cutting down on carbohydrates means that you don't eat too much fat either. Most important of all, with a low carbohydrate diet, you still get all the nutrients you need from other foods while you slim. Such a diet should enable most women to lose weight gradually and comfortably without starving themselves, and then to keep the weight off.

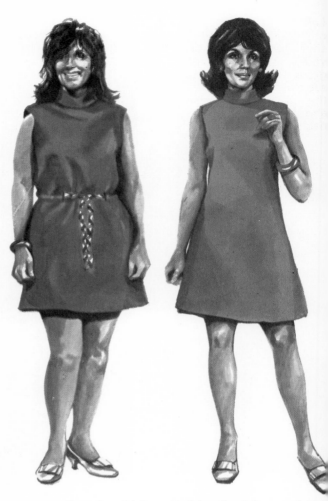

Any diet should be combined with regular exercise of an unstrenuous nature. Frequent mild exercise will help burn up extra calories and keep you from regaining weight. It will also tone muscles, improve blood circulation, and generally make you more shapely. Strenuous exercise should be avoided because it can tax your heart, especially if you are overweight, and can also stimulate appetite.

You can maintain your body in tip-top condition by keeping just three rules in mind: Do a reasonable amount of exercise; eat out of need for good health rather than for emotional reasons; and follow a generally high-protein, low-carbohydrate diet, being sure to get a full range of vitamins and minerals. This simple program will help you remain healthy, vital, and trim for your whole life long.

Left: to see yourself as others see you would be a shock for many. You see yourself as trim, well-groomed, and neat. Others see the windblown hair, the rumples you ignored, and the extra pounds you hadn't noticed at all.

Right: the walk you take with your child to give her some fresh air is good for you, too—take a few deep breaths, and enjoy being vitally alive.

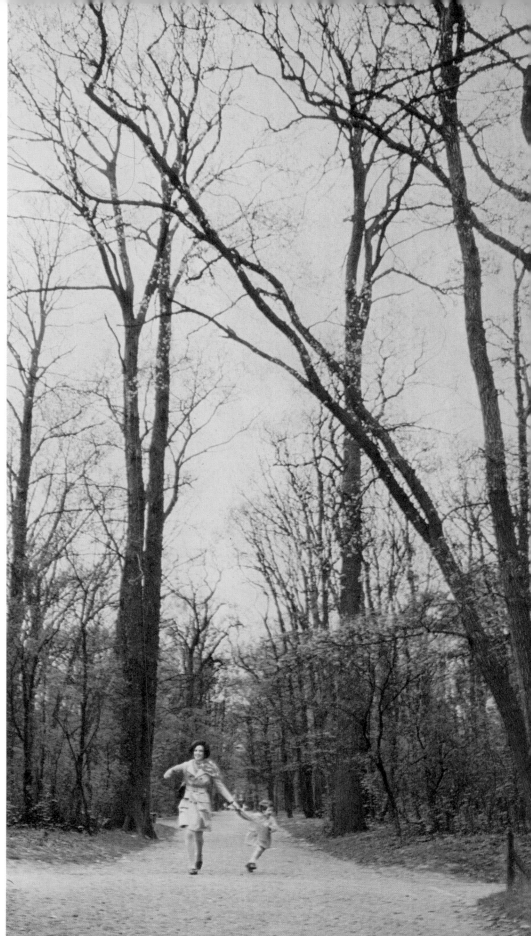

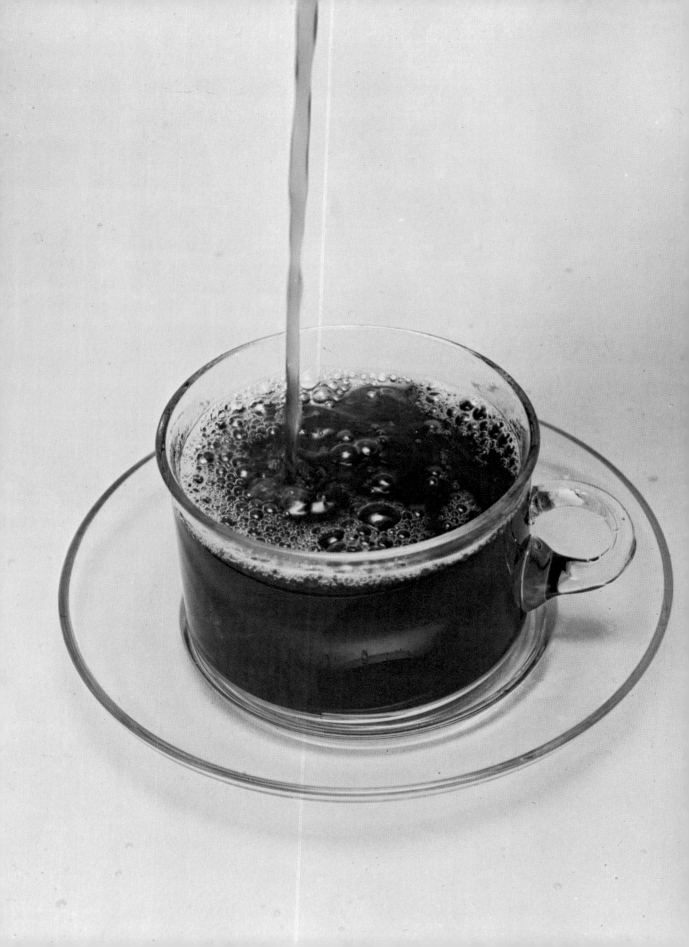

Coffee, Aspirin, and Other Poisons

5

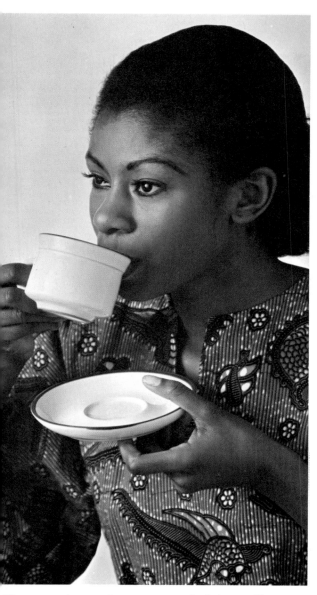

There are times when you may feel that coffee makes your world go round—especially first thing in the morning. But the very potency that coffee has to make you feel better is a sure indication of its strong effect—which may not be too good.

Nutrition is only part of the chemical story behind glowing good health. While we must take in every day the foods that keep our bodies properly functioning and in good repair, it is just as important to keep harmful chemicals out. This, however, is not so easy, for we humans have invented hundreds of concoctions to produce some desired effect or other: to pep us up, slow us down, or to relieve our real and imagined aches of body and mind. They range from foods that contain drugs, such as coffee and tea, through a variety of self-medications, to the psychic crutches such as tobacco, alcohol, stimulants and tranquilizers. These items share three things in common: most of them can be found in nearly every home; they can, when properly used, serve some useful function; and they are all potentially harmful.

Take coffee and tea—the most widely consumed beverages in the Western world. Every day Europeans and Americans brew and drink them in the tens of millions of quarts. Few would deny that a steaming cup of rich coffee is a delightful way to begin the day or top off a good dinner. And, as many women know, a coffee-break at home or in the office can help to ease the day's tasks. For some of us it seems an absolute necessity. Yet both coffee and tea contain an active drug factor—caffeine. Taken in excess caffeine can be fatal. And although doctors estimate that it would take 10 grams—more than 100 cups of coffee or tea—to kill you, just 1 gram—about 10 cups—is enough to produce such unpleasant side-effects as nausea, restlessness, and palpitations. Even two or three cups will increase heartbeat, stimulate your kidneys, and interefere with sleep.

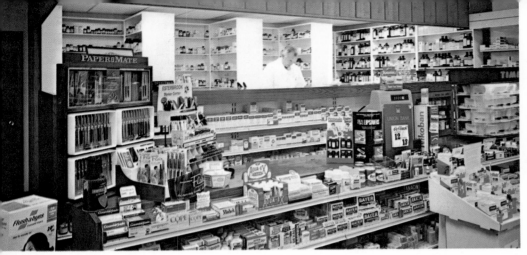

Although the law protects you by insisting that most drugs be dispensed only o prescription, it is still possible to poison yourself by stupid or absentminded use of the "harmless" medicines so readily available at the drugstore on the corner.

Right: most of these potentially dangerous items are probably lying around your house. They are especially attractive to curious young children.

1 Detergent
2 Bleach
3 Liquid Soap
4 Oven Cleaner
5 Spot Removers
6 Matches
7 Window Cleaner
8 Car Polish
9 Gasoline
10 Oil
11 Car Shampoo
12 Anti-Freeze
13 Shampoo
14 Hair Spray
15 After Shave
16 Rubbing Alcohol
17 Medicines
18 Disinfectant
19 Cosmetics
20 Moth Balls
21 Oral Contraceptives
22 Sleeping Pills
23 House Plants
24 Liquor
25 Furniture Polish
26 Floor Polish
27 Wood Preservative
28 Pesticides
29 Weed Killers
30 Paint Strippers
31 Glue
32 Rat Poison

82

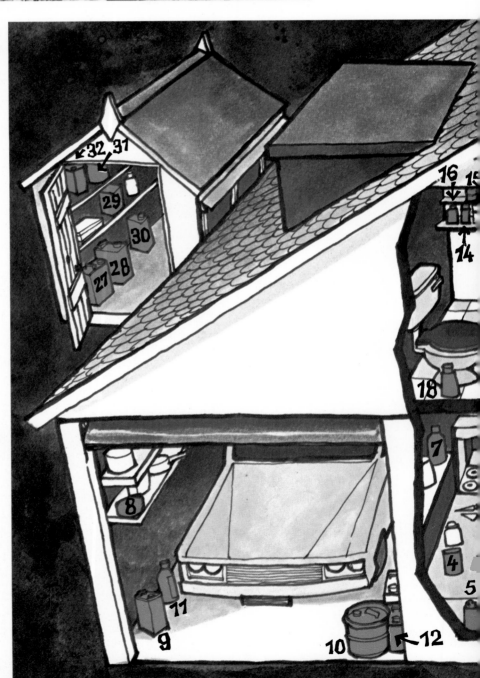

Strong doses of coffee fed to animals in laboratory tests have also been found to produce multiple B-vitamin deficiencies. This is thought to be because caffeine, by increasing the flow of blood through the kidneys, causes B-vitamins to be sent out of the kidneys in the urine. Famous American nutritionist Adelle Davis says that "heavy coffee drinkers invariably show symptoms of B-vitamin deficiencies even when their diet (otherwise) is excellent."

Coffee does change our body chemistry.

Otherwise it would not have the effect that we like. And the same goes for tea, since a cup of tea contains as much caffeine as a cup of coffee. But this does not mean that you should abstain from these drinks, or that moderate coffee or tea-drinking will necessarily interfere with your health. On the other hand, it is clear that large amounts of coffee or tea are harmful, and any confirmed coffee or tea-lover would do well to ensure that her Vitamin-B intake exceeds the recommended minimum requirements

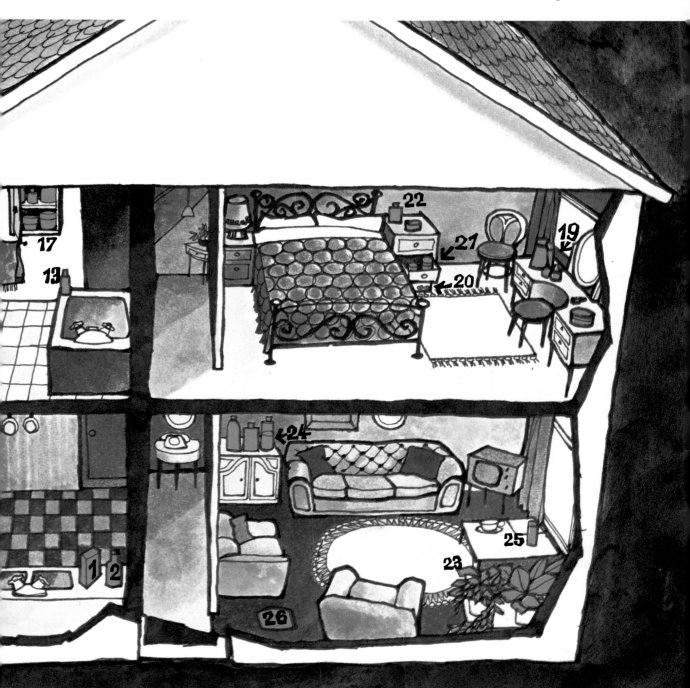

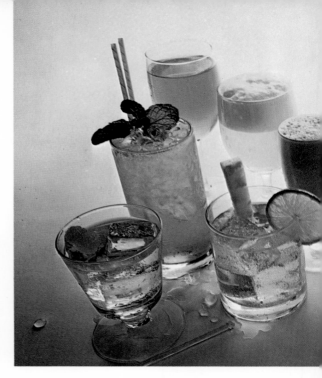

(see Chapter 4 and chart on page 66).

Aspirin is another potential poison readily at hand. It is by far the commonest of all the household remedies. No one thinks twice about taking a couple of aspirin tablets every now and then to relieve minor aches and pains. And, properly used, aspirin is indeed one of the most valuable mild pain-killers available. But aspirin, or aspirin-based medicines, should on no account be taken for an "upset stomach," or by anyone who suffers from stomach trouble, because it can cause bleeding from the stomach lining. (For this reason, it is always advisable to take aspirin with a milk chaser.) And aspirin should never be taken in more than the recommended dose. For, as the American Medical Association has warned in its journal, aspirin is a dangerous drug if our diets do not contain enough Vitamin C to detoxify it. This vitamin, while preventing aspirin from poisoning our system, is itself destroyed. Thus, each aspirin we take robs the body of a certain amount of the Vitamin C needed for important bodily functions. And the more tablets we swallow, the more risk we run of reaching a point where there is no Vitamin C available to detoxify the drug, and acute aspirin poisoning will occur.

Aspirin overdose is one of the commonest forms of accidental death. Fifteen to twenty aspirin tablets taken over a 24-hour period can be fatal to an adult. Ten or twelve tablets taken in one gulp may do the same job quicker. Aspirin deaths often occur among children who get into the family medicine chest. In other cases, aspirin overdose may result from an excessive reliance on the tablets for the relief of every-

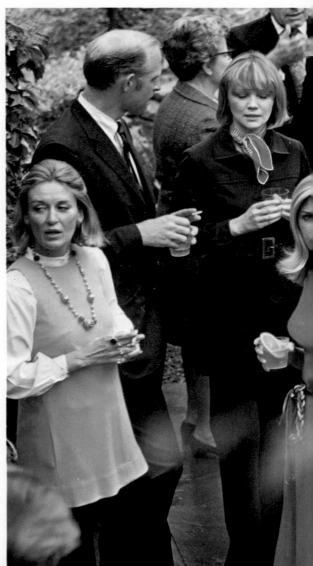

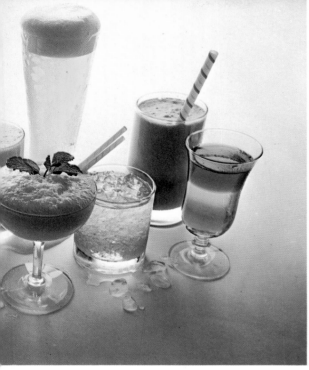

Drinking is a pleasant, relaxing part of our social pattern. For many people it never becomes more. But for some, alchohol becomes such a necessary drug that drinking for them is a hopeless addiction.

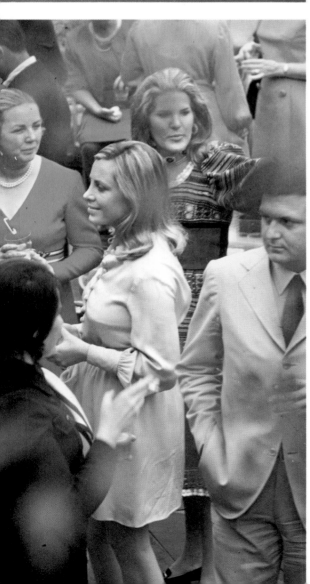

day stresses. Aspirin does have a mild tranquilizing effect, and this is one of the reasons why it is so useful for combating occasional irritating ills, like headaches, from which we all suffer. But some people get into the habit of taking a few aspirin tablets regularly whenever they feel anxious, ache a little, or cannot sleep. After continued regular use, more and more tablets are needed to obtain relief, and a person may work herself up to a fatal dose without even realizing it.

Aspirin is not a universal remedy. There are some kinds of physical pain or severe stress which may not be reduced by the drug. So, if you find that the standard dose of two aspirins does not help, the sensible course is to ask a physician about a different pain-relieving drug.

Other so-called harmless drugs sold over the counter in the drug store are also frequently abused, few more so than laxatives. Many people are still wrongly convinced that a daily bowel movement is the single most important gauge of health. If a day goes by without elimination, worry often leads them to give nature a helping hand with a dose of this or that. But doctors assure us that the necessity of a daily bowel movement is a myth. Just as in the case of menstruation, people vary in this respect. The large intestine differs in size and activity according to the individual, and this results in different requirements and rhythms. Failure to empty the bowel does not cause disease, since poisonous products in the bowel cannot be absorbed into the system. As proof of this, one doctor cites the case of a man who did not have a bowel movement

85

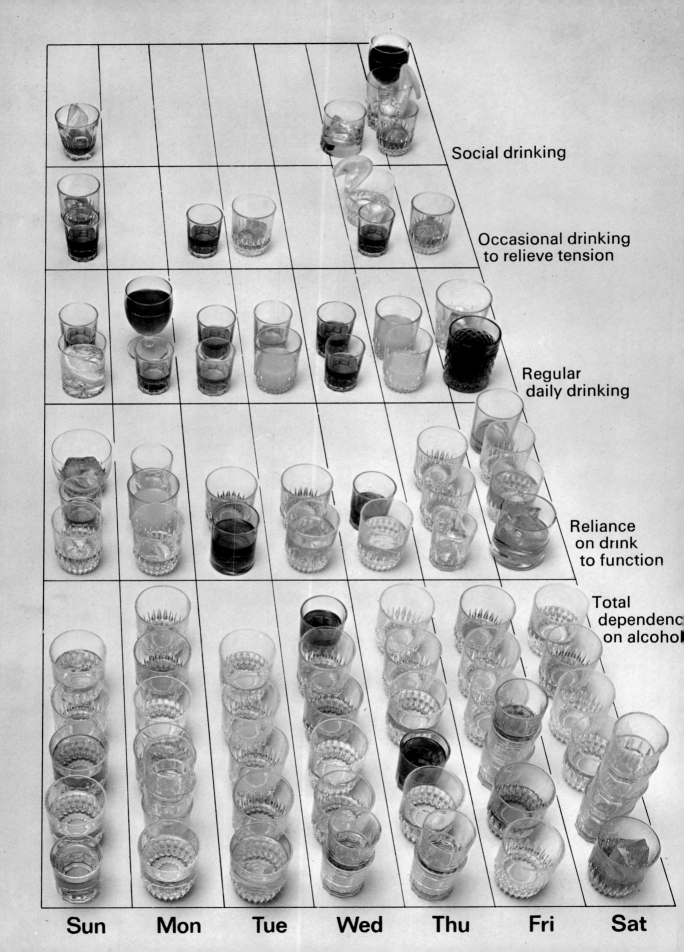

Social drinking

Occasional drinking to relieve tension

Regular daily drinking

Reliance on drink to function

Total dependence on alcohol

Sun **Mon** **Tue** **Wed** **Thu** **Fri** **Sat**

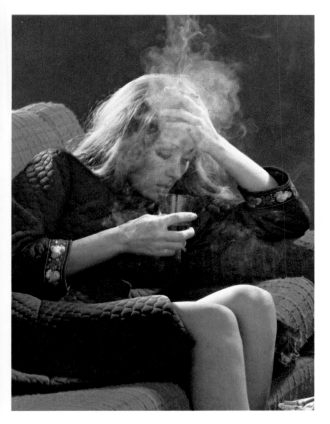

Far left: in relation to drinking, where would you place yourself on this chart? If you added up what you drank last week, you might find that it's more than you thought. That doesn't mean you're slipping into dependency, but it is a signal for caution. Below: alcoholism is not a rare disease, either among women or men. This chart shows the number of women alcoholics by age per 10,000 population.

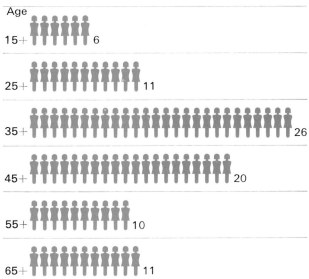

Age		
15+	🚶🚶🚶🚶🚶🚶	6
25+	🚶🚶🚶🚶🚶🚶🚶🚶🚶🚶🚶	11
35+	🚶🚶🚶🚶🚶🚶🚶🚶🚶🚶🚶🚶🚶🚶🚶🚶🚶🚶🚶🚶🚶🚶🚶🚶🚶🚶	26
45+	🚶🚶🚶🚶🚶🚶🚶🚶🚶🚶🚶🚶🚶🚶🚶🚶🚶🚶🚶🚶	20
55+	🚶🚶🚶🚶🚶🚶🚶🚶🚶🚶	10
65+	🚶🚶🚶🚶🚶🚶🚶🚶🚶🚶🚶	11

for a whole year and was not in the least ill—although his abdomen was somewhat swollen.

Obviously few of us would want to experience what that man did, for, even if constipation does not make us ill, it can make us feel uncomfortable. But if the daily bowel movement is not a guide, what exactly constitutes constipation? The answer again varies with the individual. Each person has his or her own pattern of regularity, but as a general rule, doctors say that you are constipated if you have not had a bowel movement for about three days.

The best treatment for constipation is a change in diet. Eating more green vegetables, plenty of fresh and stewed fruits, and other foods that contain roughage, such as bran and oatmeal cereals, will help. And you should try to drink about two quarts of liquid a day, preferably water or diluted fruit juices. Milk or milk-based drinks, on the other hand, tend to have a constipating effect. It is also helpful to establish a regular time each day to have a bowel movement.

Failing all this, there is no harm in taking an occasional dose of a mild laxative. But over-reliance on laxatives should be avoided at all costs. Laxatives can have a number of harmful effects, and, in some cases, may even increase constipation. Continual use of laxatives can make the bowel lazy so that it will not perform its natural task on its own.

Some laxatives stimulate bowel action with irritating substances. Overuse of these products can result in a highly-inflamed large intestine. Other laxatives are based on mineral oils that lubricate the lower bowel to allow waste material to move through it more easily. While these laxatives perform their job fairly effectively, they, too, have the effect of making the lower intestine lazy. Mineral oil preparations can also prevent the absorption of oil soluble vitamins. Continual use may thus result in deficiencies of Vitamins A, D, E, and K.

For the treatment of minor, easily recognized complaints, home medicines can be

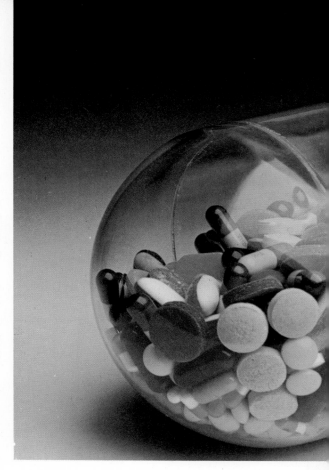

valuable aids, provided they are used only occasionally and in the doses recommended on the bottle. But all self-medications are dangerous when used to excess.

Perhaps the most dangerous drink that we humans have invented is alcohol. Alcohol is a drug. Taken in excess it can kill. Used in moderate amounts, its effects are pleasant and harmless. As with all drugs, its effect depends on how you use it.

Alcoholic content varies widely from drink to drink. Beer is relatively weak in alcohol. Wine may be twice as strong, and hard liquor, such as gin, whiskey, rum, brandy or vodka, may contain more than 40 per cent alcohol. Different people react differently to the same amount of alcohol, and this is why it is impossible to lay down precisely what is a "safe" amount to drink. For legal purposes, however, some limit often has to be set, notably to control drunken driving. But one thing is certain. Even the smallest glass of any alcoholic drink affects the delicately balanced functioning of your body.

Most women know that a glass or two of wine, a cocktail, an ounce or two of whiskey, or a couple of cans of good beer produce a temporary sense of warmth and well-being. The alcohol in these drinks dilates the blood vessels of the skin and brings an increased flow of warm blood to the skin surfaces. The pleasant relaxation and sense of well-being is created because alcohol depresses the central nervous system. It acts as an anesthetic on the cerebral cortex which exercises conscious control over behavior. With the cortex lulled into happy lassitude, the primitive brain has a freer rein. So if you brighten up after a drink, or speak and act just a trifle more freely than usual, you do so because the restraining influences which usually monitor behavior have been diminished. Several drinks can dull perception of feelings and surroundings, diminish self-criticism and the fear of actions which we might usually regard as inappropriate—if not downright impolite or uncivilized. This gradual lessening of inhibitions may make you more amorous, sentimental, or even depressed. It all depends on your basic character and, to some extent, on your mood at the time.

The more you drink, the greater is the effect of alcohol on the nervous system. This eventually disturbs balance, so that the drinker begins to stagger and fumble and may pass out. A still higher concentration of alcohol will depress the part of the brain that controls breathing. This lethal level is generally reckoned to be equivalent to about eight or nine large whiskies or other spirits.

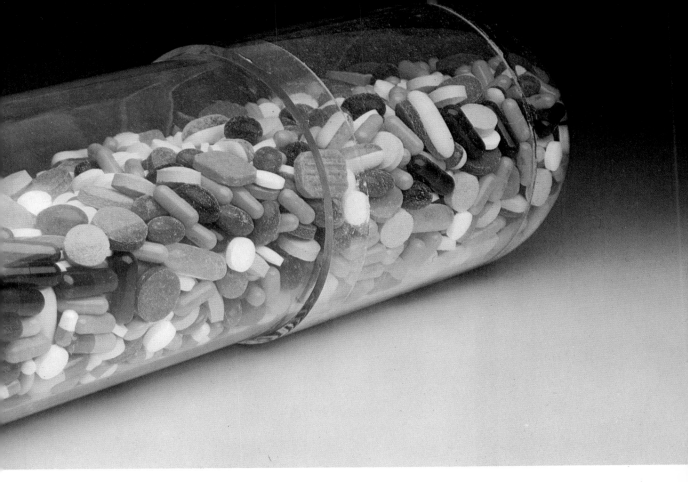

Apart from its action on the nervous system, alcohol also raises the rate of urine production. But only about two per cent of the alcohol drunk will escape in the urine and, in the meantime, the body cells gradually become dehydrated. This is what causes the sensation of thirst and the dry, furry tongue of a typical hangover. Doctors advise anyone who wants to combat these after-effects to drink about a pint of water after a party. The other main symptom of a hangover, an upset stomach, is caused because alcohol irritates the delicate lining of the stomach, making it produce excess acid. This effect is reduced when food is taken with drink or before drinking. Food protects the stomach-lining and slows down absorption of alcohol into the bloodstream. Milk or milk-drinks taken before a party have the same effect and also help to neutralize stomach acid.

Once alcohol has entered the bloodstream, it quickly passes into all the tissues and fluids of the body. Moderate amounts of alcohol are then detoxified, or rendered harmless, by the liver. The problem occurs, however, when the amount of alcohol taken in exceeds the capacity of the liver to detoxify it. Then it starts killing cells, starting with the liver. So-called cirrhosis of the liver is the progressive destruction of liver tissue and its replacement by scar tissue. As the liver is slowly destroyed, its ability to detoxify alcohol diminishes. Progressively less alcohol is required to exceed the liver's capacity, and it takes less alcohol, rather than more, to produce intoxication. After liver cells, next in susceptibility to alcohol are nerve cells, including those of the brain. Alcohol damages the protective cell membranes and crosses into the cells where it can upset the chemical balance and finally destroy them.

Contrary to popular mythology, the most serious health problem of alcoholics is neither cirrhosis nor brain damage, but malnu-

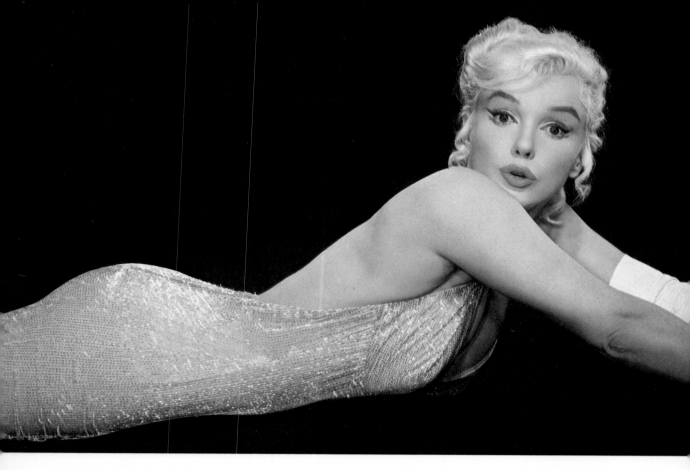

Above: death from an overdose of sleeping pills catches public attention when it involves a celebrity, such as spectacular Hollywood star Marilyn Monroe. However, thousands of ordinary people in the crowd die every year from the same cause.

trition. Since alcohol tends to diminish the appetite for food and deaden the sense of taste, the alcoholic eats less and less food and relies almost entirely on alcohol for energy. This in turn, leads to malnutrition and a lower resistance to diseases.

According to the American Mental Health Association, there are more than four million known alcoholics in the United States— one million of them women. Alcoholics Anonymous estimates that there are 80,000 women alcoholics in New York City alone. And authorities agree that tens of thousands more women are secret or borderline alcoholics.

How does a woman become an alcoholic? Research has shown that such a woman usually begins drinking at parties or other social functions in order to overcome shy-

ness and join in the fun. Or she finds that a drink helps ease the strain of her job or home life, or of loneliness. Once she discovers that drinking offers a positive relief from her tensions, she then starts using it more regularly to escape from the hard realities of her world.

Soon it may seem quite a good idea to take one tiny drink to get the day's work started, maybe another to put her in the right frame of mind for a particular chore and then another small drink or two at night in order to go to sleep. She is never drunk at any point, but merely feels much more efficient, happy, and relaxed. Her drinking seems so obviously beneficial that she cannot see any harm in it. But by this stage she is quite probably becoming psychologically dependent on alcohol. The next and final step, of course, is when she can no longer operate without alcohol. She has become physically addicted.

It is the opinion of Arthur Fisher, an American researcher in the field of alco-

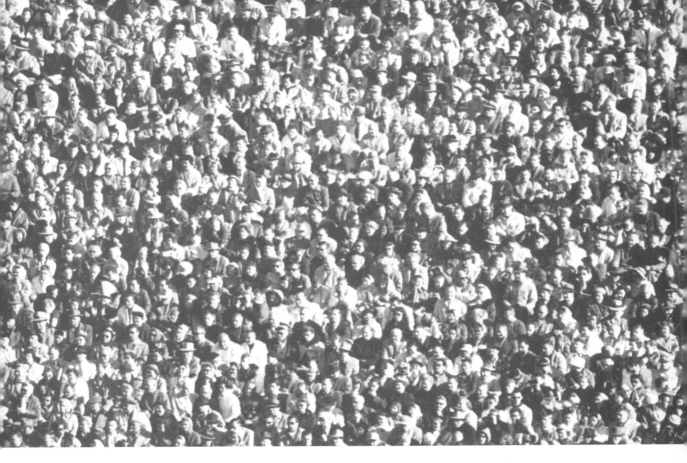

holism and drug addiction that, in both cases, the same psychological predisposition exists —an inability to cope with stress. Why do some women become addicted to drugs rather than alcohol? In most cases, it seems to be because they have their first experience with narcotics at a time of emotional need and find the gratification and escape that they seek is more complete and immediate. It can happen so easily.

Take the case of an overweight woman who wants to lose her excess poundage but cannot face the discipline of a nutritionally sound, long-term diet. She feels that she cannot live with her problem any longer and she wants to lose weight in a hurry.

This woman may well ask her doctor for "water pills" to help her reduce. These pills stimulate urine production and every pint of urine is a pound of weight. But urine also carries out of the body minerals that must be replaced. Continued use of "water pills" may result in severe potassium deficiency, and potassium deficiency has the effect of causing

muscular weakness. At this point the now-slimmer woman may find herself in a continual state of exhaustion. She is tired both physically and mentally.

Because of this, she may return to her doctor—or visit another one—to get a prescription for some kind of "pick-me-up". Now she may find herself using a drug called amphetamine as a stimulant. Amphetamines give the wanted results in a hurry. They produce a delightful feeling of mental alertness and physical energy. But they also increase tension and make deep restful sleep elusive if not impossible. At this point, the woman may go to her doctor again for something to help her relax. Or she may "borrow" a few sleeping pills from a friend. These pills are likely to be barbiturates. Now the woman is caught in a vicious cycle, alternating between her "up" on amphetamines and her "down" on barbiturates.

Amphetamines and barbiturates have a legitimate use in medicine. But such drugs

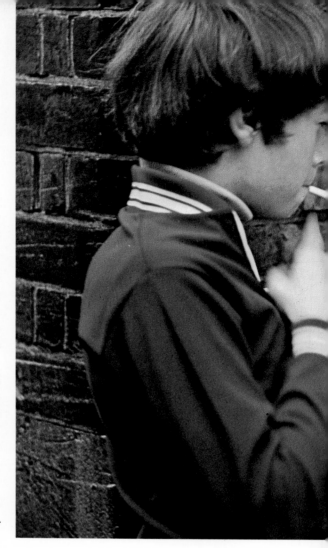

Right: for far too many teenagers, a cigarette represents sophistication. Its glamour as a sign of adulthood is much more visible than its deadly threat to good health.

should never be taken without medical supervision by a physician who knows your entire case history and also all about the kind and number of pills that you might already be taking. Yet many women continue to use amphetamines, barbiturates and other mind-affecting drugs without a doctor's prescription. Just as bad, many women take more than the dosage prescribed for them.

A recent survey has shown that 45 per cent of American women use drugs. And although less women than men use such illegal drugs as marijuana, heroin, cocaine, or LSD, far more women than men regularly take barbiturates, tranquilizers, and pep pills. These drugs are perfectly legal and "respectable," but abuse, that is excessive use, of many of them can lead to addiction.

Far and away the most dangerous of these drugs, according to many physicians, are barbiturates. Barbiturate abuse brings psychological dependence and increased tolerance. The continued use of large doses leads to physical dependence. And withdrawal from barbiturates is even more harrowing than from heroin. It usually continues for about two weeks, while the patient undergoes agonizing mental and physical suffering, and may die from convulsions or from exhaustion. Even under medical supervision, complete withdrawal may take as long as two months.

Even discounting the hazards of withdrawal, barbiturate abuse is extremely dangerous. Unintentional overdose, which is often fatal, may occur very easily. If someone takes a regular dose to go to sleep and then remains awake, or awakens shortly thereafter, she may be so confused that she will continue to take repeated normal doses. This can lead to severe poisoning or death. Fatal reactions are also possible if barbiturates and alcohol are mixed. Each drug reinforces the depressant or toxic effect of the other. Every year in the United States there are some 3,000 deaths from barbiturate overdose, accidental or intentional—more than from any other drug.

"Warning: The Surgeon General Has Determined that Cigarette Smoking is Dangerous To Your Health." This legend is printed on every package of cigarettes sold in America. What more is there to say? Except, perhaps, that if we are talking about hazards to the health of normal women, all other drugs run far behind tobacco as a *potential* cause of death. Lung cancer kills over 50,000 Americans annually, more than

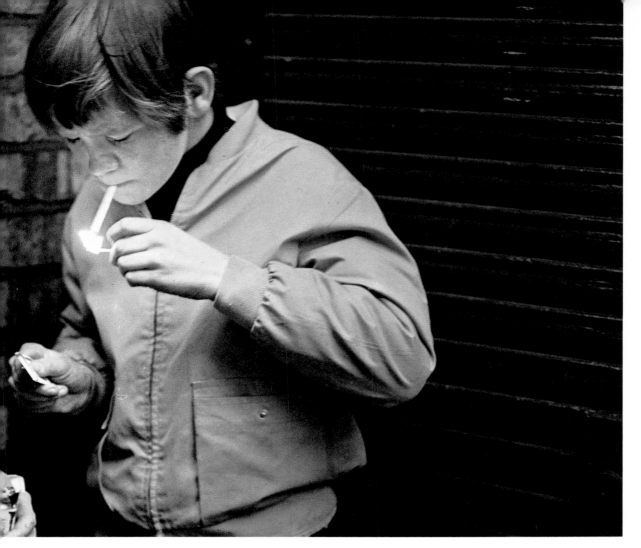

80 per cent of whom are cigarette smokers. Cigarette smoking is also believed by physicians to be the single most important cause of emphysema (a disease that decreases the efficiency of the lungs), which kills over 15,000 persons a year. Approximately 100,000 cigarette smokers die from heart attacks. Besides these horrifying numbers, there is extremely good evidence assembled by the National Institute of Health, the center of federally supported research in America, relating smoking to other circulatory diseases such as high blood pressure, as well as stomach ulcers, and cancer of the bladder. The cigarette related death toll is highest among men, but each passing year sees an increase in the number of tobacco-addicted women among the grisly statistics.

If good health is your goal, all you need to put into your body is nutritious food—and not too much of that. And when things go wrong, the U.S. Public Health Service offers these guidelines:

Self-prescribed drugs should never be used continuously for long periods of time ... a physician is required for: abdominal pain that is severe or recurs periodically; pains anywhere, if severe, disabling, persistent, or recurring; headache, if unusually severe or prolonged more than one day; a prolonged cold with fever or cough; earache; unexplained loss of weight; unexplained and unusual symptoms; *malaise* lasting more than a week or two.

Your body is indeed a fantastic machine. It is, for the most part, self-repairing and self-regulating. But to keep it well, you must treat it well.

93

Feel Fit, Look Good!

6

Advertisements in our newspapers, magazines, and on commercial television programs hawk beauty as if it were a commodity. They shout and implore: "buy this lotion, use that shampoo, paint your eyes with cosmetic X, drink this, wear that, and you will be beautiful." What the advertisements don't tell us is that the single most important element of beauty is health. True beauty cannot be bought or painted on. It comes from feeling good inside. When you glow with health, you look good and you make the people around you feel good too.

Linda Clark, author of *Stay Young Longer*, says that a really vital factor in a woman's beauty is a healthy, happy inner self. Frowns are not flattering. Neither are the hard, sullen looks that so many women—and men—unconsciously assume as they go about their daily life. Expressions of boredom, weariness, and tension also frequently mar an otherwise beautiful face.

A woman shows her inner self not only in her face, but also in the way she holds herself, the way she walks, and in her reaction to the people and things around her. So, if you want to look your best, you must start your personal appearance program from the inside and work out. Aim at maintaining your body machine in top physical condition through proper eating, sensible exercise, and adequate rest. Work at reducing and managing tension. These two aspects of health go together, and if you are diligent, you can have—completely free and forever—your own intimate and personal beauty.

One essential part of any program for healthful living is daily exercise. Work alone is usually not enough, because it exercises

Right: much of the pleasure of good health is the joy of being able to use your body just as you wish, running without feeling weak, and playing without getting sore.

94

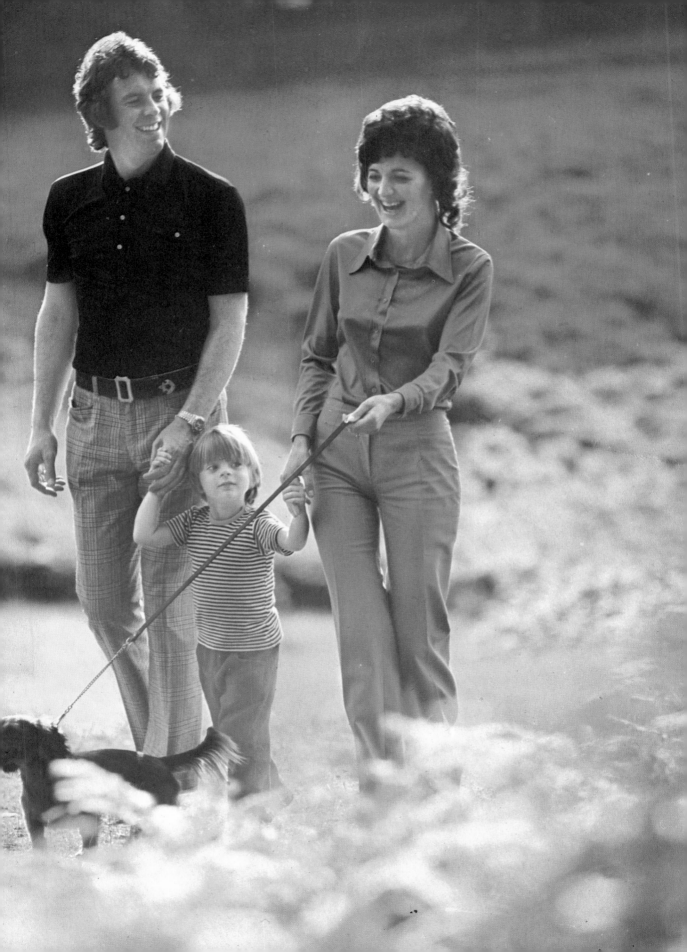

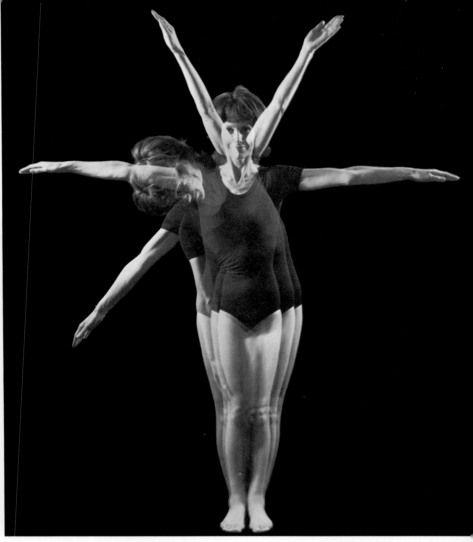

Children use every muscle in their bodies daily, so that they stay supple and limber. Adults tend to become stiffer because certain parts of the body go unused. Regular exercise—such as mild calisthenics or swimming—help keep the adult body lithe and in good shape.

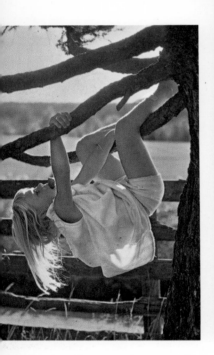

only certain muscles—and often not in the proper way. Exercising for health, however, is like eating for health. Both work best when you follow a regular regime and least well when you try to beat past abuses with crash programs. So, if you lead a sedentary life and are feeling a bit flabby, don't embark on a vigorous fitness campaign first thing tomorrow. The most you will get from a sudden bout of strenuous exercise is a lot of sore muscles and the resolve to give the whole thing up. Instead, make it a rule to do at least 10 minutes mild exercise each day. Small amounts of exercise do mount up, and a minimal exercise program is enough to keep you fit, healthy and vital—provided you follow it regularly.

Regular exercise pays plenty of dividends. It improves blood circulation and brings a glow to your skin. By toning up muscles, it helps fight flab and dispels the aches and pains that come from bad posture. Experiments have shown that exercise keeps your heart and lungs in good shape and decreases the risk of heart disease. It is also believed to stimulate the hormone-producing glands which are so important to emotional and physical well-being. Exercise helps you to overcome fatigue and tension, and may even improve digestion, for, as Thomas Cureton of the University of Illinois Physical Fitness Laboratory says, "even the best of foods cannot be assimilated without exercise."

Remember that you can't count on exercise to get rid of excess poundage. Diet first. But once you have lost the fat, exercise is just as important as diet in weight control. If you add exercise to a moderate diet, the

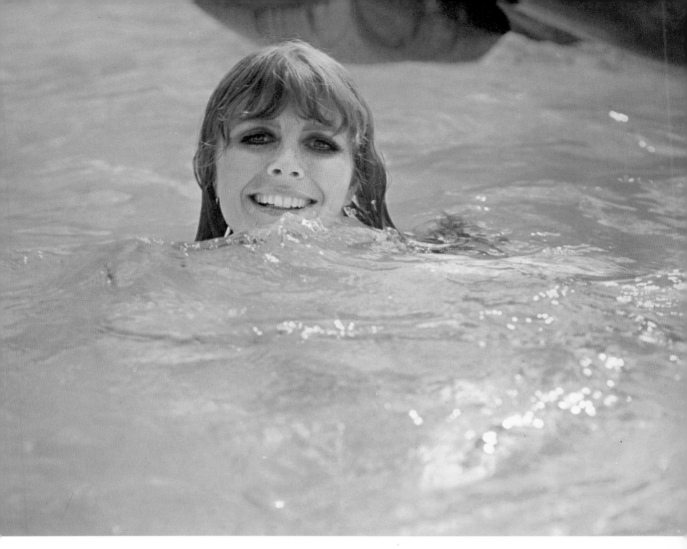

extra minutes of activity will help you keep weight off and reeducate lax muscles to give you a better shape. As leading figure expert Lotte Berk, now a trim and shapely 58-year-old, says, "If you exercise regularly, you will never lose your figure, whatever your age, and you will never have to wear elasticated girdles or corsets. Your own muscles will hold you in shape."

So what sort of exercise should you take? The answer depends largely on your own temperament. "One of the most important findings of the new exercise methods," says Dr. Clement Martin in his *Managing Your Health,* "is that useful activity must be enjoyable if it is really going to work." He advises that a strong element of rhythm be included in whatever form of exercise you choose, and he particularly recommends swimming. Swimming has the essential rhythmic quality that many more strenuous exercises lack. And it has the added advantage that you can take the whole family along to join in the fun. To get the best out of swimming, experts advise that you should swim steadily for at least five minutes. Begin with as many lengths of the pool as you can make without exhausting yourself. Then add one lap each time you swim.

Sports, like tennis, badminton, golf, or ping-pong, also provide very good exercise, and bike-riding will help strengthen muscles. Another activity that combines exercise with pleasure is especially recommended by figure experts—dancing. Dancing, like swimming, has the rhythm that helps you control your body, acquire good balance,

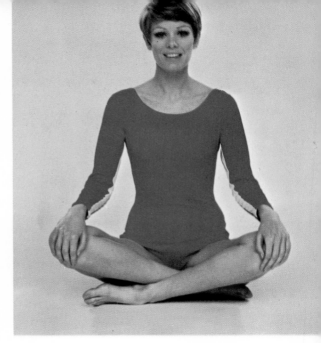

An increasingly popular system of exercising is yoga, which aims equally at developing a vigorous body and a serene mind. Yoga exercises are all done slowly, and often one position is held for a few seconds of count.

walk gracefully, and feel more relaxed. You can, of course, dance at home to a record or music on the radio. Or try taking dance lessons—tap dancing, ballet, old-time, modern, folk or flamenco, whichever appeals to you.

Walking is one exercise that most of us can probably fit into our daily routine. Strolling around the shops won't help much, but a good fast walk at least once a day is very good for your health. You should walk briskly, with rhythmic strides from the hips. Wear your most comfortable shoes and, if possible, carry only a light bag, so that you can swing your arms freely. If you have to carry heavy shopping, try to distribute the weight evenly in two bags, one for each hand. While you walk, try to keep your mind on pleasant things—a movie you have seen, or a plan for your next free week-end. Concentrated thinking can make you hunch your shoulders and tense your muscles.

Try to walk as often as you can over short distances, instead of using the car or taking the bus. And walk upstairs instead of using the elevator. This exercise, which is likely to make most of us puff and pant a bit if we are out of condition, is one of the best ways of making the whole body work as it should.

If you prefer to exercise at home, you could make a start with the 10 basic exercises that are shown beginning on page 102. And when you want a bit more variety, there are plenty of exercise programs to choose from. A very good plan, available as a book, is the one compiled by the Royal Canadian Air Force especially for modern women—and men—who lead sedentary lives

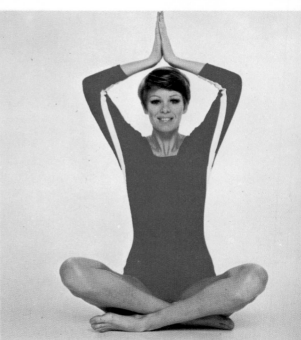

and are worried about their figures and their health, but haven't the time or the enthusiasm for active sports. Although these exercises were originally designed to keep Air Force personnel in the peak of condition, they are graded in easy stages to help you get fit and stay fit at your own pace. They begin by working on the parts of the body that are likely to have grown a bit rusty,

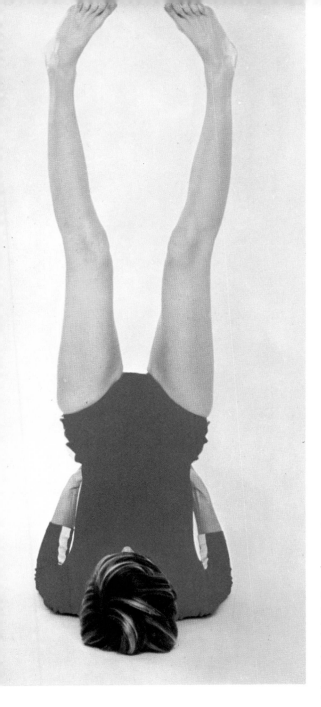

put quite a strain on the heart, particularly if you haven't done any exercise for a long time, and it is always advisable to have a physical checkup before you begin a jogging program. If you do decide on jogging—and it can be fun—you could try the program recommended by Dr. Vogin Smoldlaka of New York City. He suggests alternating 30 seconds each of running and walking, not to exceed five minutes a day to start with and gradually increasing the time.

The ancient Indian science of yoga is another way of exercising which has become increasingly popular in the West. Yoga movements and yoga breathing are intended to ease nervous tension as well as to tone muscles and to build a supple, well-poised body. One of the best things about yoga is that the exercises are smooth, graceful, and controlled. There is no strenuous jerking or breathless speed, and the exercises are never tiring. This makes yoga particularly suitable for women of all ages, and even, in many cases, for those whose health otherwise prevents strenuous activity. Yoga expert Richard Hittleman, who has done a lot to promote the study of yoga in the United States and Europe, says that he regularly has pupils from ages 4 to over 80 exercising in his yoga classes.

Here is just one simple yoga exercise for you to try to see how you like it: Sit on the floor with your legs stretched straight out in front of you and your feet together. Very slowly, stretch out your arms until they are parallel with your legs, and then raise them in slow motion up and back. Lean back several inches and then slowly come forward, bending your body toward your legs. Slide

and progress to exercises that concentrate on specific areas—waistline, bottom, thighs, and so on. Best of all, perhaps, they take only a few minutes each day.

Jogging—a combination of running and walking—is one of the newest exercises which has many advocates. But jogging can be dangerous. It may cause torn ligaments and muscles, as well as sore feet. Jogging can also

your hands down your legs and curl your hands round your knees, lower legs, ankles or feet—whichever you can reach comfortably. Gently move your trunk downward, bending your elbows outward as you go, getting your forehead as near your knees as you can without strain. Hold the position for a count of 5. Then, very slowly straighten up and relax.

If you like the feel of yoga, you can learn a lot from Richard Hittleman's books on the subject. But, although you can study yoga at home, it does take time and practice to learn well, and you will make more rapid progress by taking classes from a master teacher.

By contrast, isometric exercises offer a modern approach to the problem of tightening flabby muscles. Isometrics are particularly good as an addition to a general fitness program, since they enable you to concentrate on the particular group of muscles you want to tone up—a sagging bust, waistline, or bottom, for example—without wasting energy on the others. Isometrics work by using groups of muscles to pull or push against a resisting object. To strengthen waist, diaphragm and stomach muscles, for example, you hold the sides of the chair in which you are sitting and push hard as if you were trying to force the chair through the floor, and then relax. For thigh and bottom muscles, you simply pull the buttocks together as hard as you can to a count of 10 and then relax. One big advantage of isometrics is that many of the simpler exercises are quick to do and can often be practiced at odd moments during the day. But some more advanced isometric exer-

cises that are designed to build muscle size can be very hard work indeed.

Whatever the program you choose, make sure that the exercises appeal to you enough to make you feel that you can face doing them regularly—and that they are right for your age, weight and degree of fitness. In general, vigorous exercises that depend a great deal on speed are best for the under twenty-fives. Advanced muscle-building programs, needing strength, may suit those in their late twenties, but are more likely to appeal to budding Mr. Universes than to women. Endurance exercises that use the heart and lungs, like running and walking, are normally suitable at any age. Mobility exercises that work each joint through its full range of movement are good for all age-groups.

More important than age, however, is the question of how fit you are and how ready your heart and muscles are to take on a little extra work. Some women in their twenties and thirties are a good deal less active than grandmothers in their sixties and seventies. And sedentary living gradually decreases the efficiency of all body systems, not just muscles. That is why it is so important not to plunge straight from lethargy into vigorous exercise. You should be especially careful to get your doctor's permission for exercising if you are at all overweight. Any extra weight means extra strain on the heart, and even a toe-touching exercise can endanger the spine as it strains to lift a heavy torso.

Many doctors claim that women are often stronger and fitter after the birth of children, and of course exercises are now an important

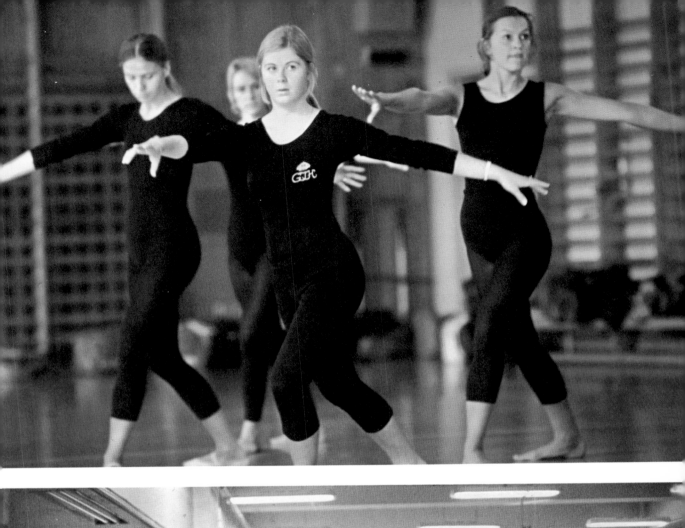
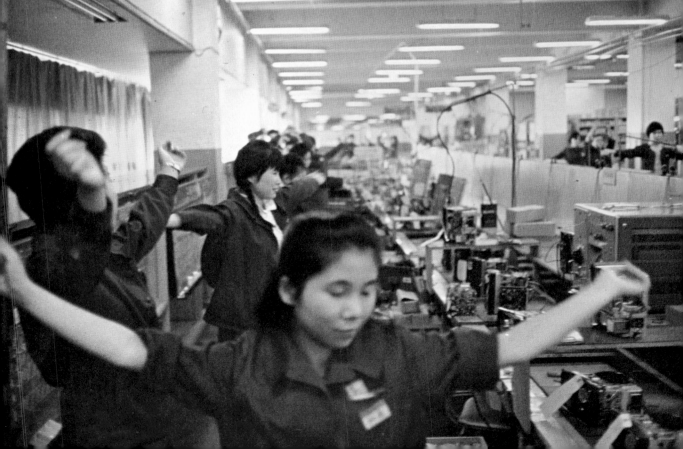

part of postnatal, as well as prenatal fitness. But doctors advise women against any exercise that involves heavy lifting. And if you have any sort of internal operation, you should not do exercises that involve lying on your back and raising your legs. All women should avoid exercises that give any pain in the small of the back. And never do push-ups. Push-ups are great for young men. But, since a woman's body is built quite differently, these exercises could make you round-shouldered and flat-chested, as well as giving you a protruding stomach.

The best way of checking whether your exercise program is right for your individual needs is to consult your doctor. And, unless you are absolutely sure that your health is reasonably sound, don't embark on any exercise program whatever without your doctor's advice. Remember to exercise gently at first, and in time your body will adjust to the new demands being made on it.

You can exercise anywhere, but many experts believe that privacy is best. They want you to really feel your body at work, to huff and puff as you need to, and to enjoy exercising without inhibition. A musical background will help you keep up a comfortable rhythm. Choose the tune to suit your pace, and music will make exercising much more fun.

Do your exercises whenever you can snatch the time. Before breakfast is the ideal moment—if you can bear it. Busy mothers may find that they have to bring their children in on the act, but that doesn't matter—they will think it's a great game. Whatever the moment you choose, however, do wait for at least an hour after a meal, or indigestion may spoil all the good work you're doing.

Whatever the experts say, many women find it more encouraging to work with others in an exercise class. This can help boost flagging will-power and turn exercising into a pleasant social event. And there is no need to worry about looking foolish. If you feel lumpy and self-conscious, so does everybody else. And another big plus in

A daily routine doing the following 10 basic exercises will improve your physical fitness immensely, helping you to release tensions, fight tiredness, and keep your heart and lungs in good shape. These easy exercises will also help you keep your figure in good shape by fighting flabbiness. Start by doing each exercise only once, and increase the number of times as it becomes easier for you. Don't exercise on a full stomach—and try putting on a favorite record and working out in rhythm to it.

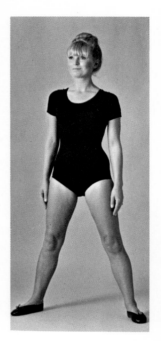

Downward Swing. Stand with legs apart (left) raise your arms, and then swing them down and touch the floor between your feet (right). Do this four times, and bend knees if necessary.

Below: Side Swing. Stand with legs apart, arms raised, hands clasped. Swing down and touch your right foot with your clasped hands. Bend in the knees if you have to at first. Do three times, then repeat on left side.

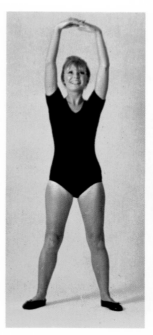

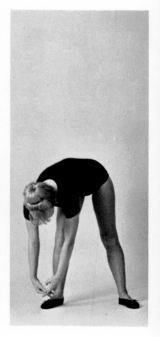

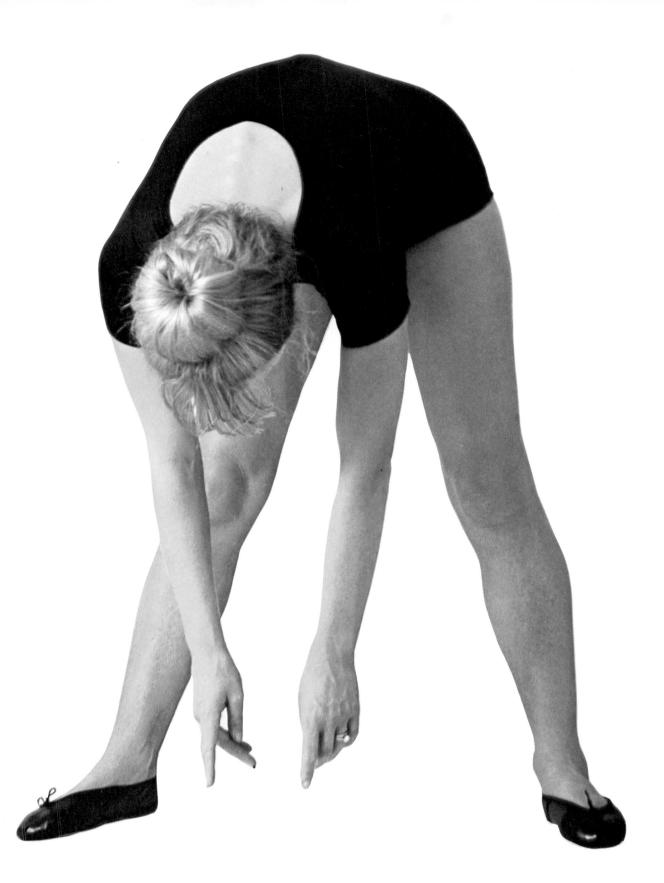

103

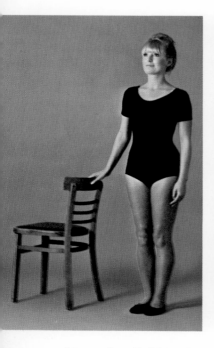 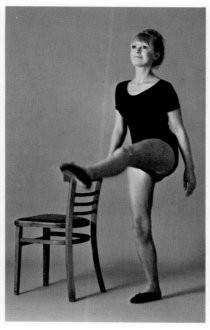 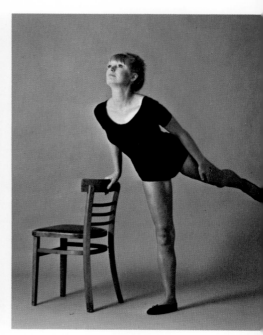

Above: Leg Raising. Stand beside a chair, placing your hand on the back of it. Raise your right leg up until it is parallel with the floor, keeping it straight. Do this twice, then raise your leg behind your back twice, as high as you can, keeping it straight. Bend the rest of your body as far forward as needed. Do twice; then repeat with the left leg.

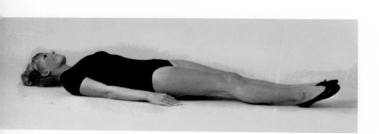

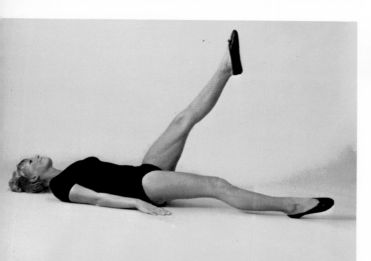

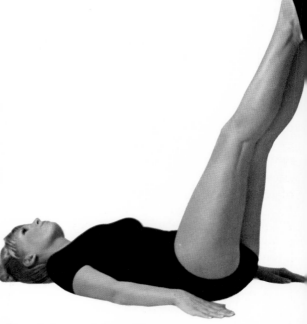

Left and above: Scissor Movement. Lie down flat on the floor. Raise one leg, then the other one, then both at the same time. Raise them as high as you can without straining, keeping the knees straight. Do this twice. (CAUTION: leave out this exercise if you have had any kind of internal operation).

exercise classes is that you can get sympathetic advice on how best to deal with your own particular figure problems.

Most of us have one particular part of our body that we'd like to change for the better. Can it be done? The answer is yes. But there are limits. Your basic skeleton cannot be altered. You have only fat and muscles to work with, and, unfortunately, you cannot take the fat off just in one spot. Fat is lost by burning more calories than you consume and it comes off all parts of the body at the same time. Muscle, however, can be built up selectively to make you a better shape.

Suppose, for example, a woman has pleasantly proportioned legs, but heavy buttocks and waist. What does she do? First she should go on a diet to get rid of the extra fat. But then her legs will be too skinny, because she will have lost weight there too. So, while exercising her whole body to keep it trim, she should concentrate on leg exercises that will build up the muscle tissue there in order to bring her legs into proportion with her now slimmer buttocks and waist.

But there is one important exception to this rule—the bust. Breasts are composed of tissue and contain no muscle. Their size is determined by glands and exercising cannot change it. What exercises can do, however, is to tighten the muscles around the breasts to give you a firmer bustline. One such exercise, which is particularly helpful for sagging breasts, is to stretch your arms out in front of you, bend your elbows, and grip your forearms as if you were pushing up both sleeves at once. Push several times in sharp jerks, then relax. You should repeat this exercise about six times a day.

Whether your bust is too big or too small for your liking, the good posture that comes from exercising in general can also help. But no treatment, either to boost or reduce your bosom, should ever be undertaken without the advice of your doctor.

Apart from being vital to your looks and comfort, the way you stand, sit, and move is

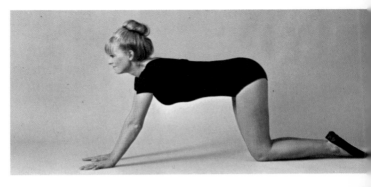

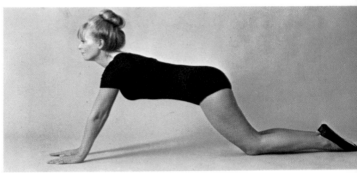

Above and below: Kneel-ups. Kneel down on the floor and place your hands on the floor in front of you. Lower yourself slowly onto your stomach, and then raise your body back to the original kneeling position once more. Repeat this exercise twice.

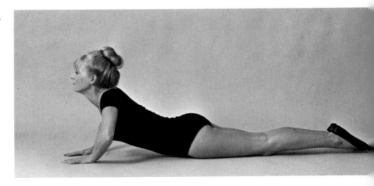

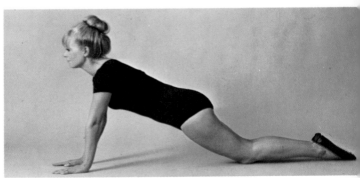

also important to your health. Good posture aids breathing, circulation, digestion and even the nervous system to function efficiently, and puts far less strain on muscles and joints.

Check your posture by taking a good look at yourself in a full-length mirror. Lift up your head and chest, and keep your shoulders well back but relaxed. Pull in your stomach muscles, gently tuck in your bottom, and tilt your pelvis slightly upward. By this time most of us tend to look a bit like tailor's dummies because we're concentrating so hard and overtensing our muscles. So it is important to remember to breathe deeply and slowly while you right your posture. Then all parts of your body will be evenly balanced but relaxed—and you will look slimmer both fore and aft. If you find that standing generally makes you tired, don't be tempted to shift from foot to foot, but place one foot in front of the other, balancing your weight evenly between the two.

For sitting, it is best to keep your behind well back in the chair and your spine straight but relaxed, with your stomach muscles held in as firmly as possible. And when you are walking, point your feet straight forward with the weight on the outside. If you turn your feet outward or inward, you will upset the balance of your body, putting a strain on your muscles and the circulation in your feet.

Making the right moves as you go about your daily chores is also important. When dusting furniture, for example, you should bend your knees and put your weight on the balls of your feet, placing one foot in front of the other to balance weight, and keeping

106

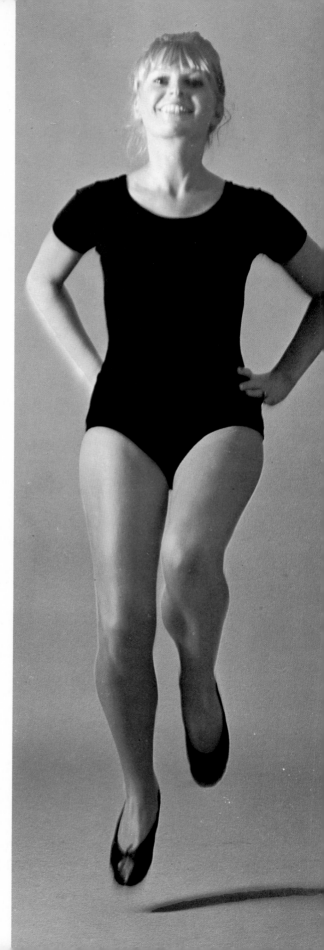

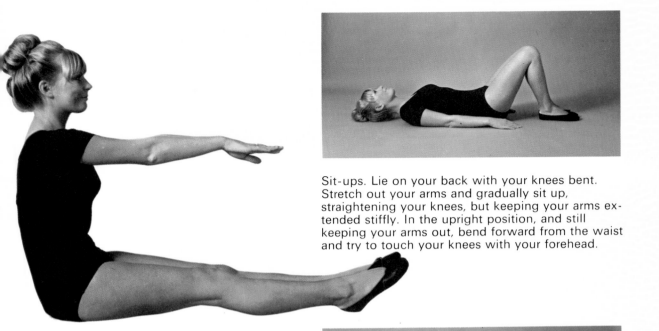

Sit-ups. Lie on your back with your knees bent. Stretch out your arms and gradually sit up, straightening your knees, but keeping your arms extended stiffly. In the upright position, and still keeping your arms out, bend forward from the waist and try to touch your knees with your forehead.

Left: Spot Running. Run lightly 20 times without moving from the same spot. You will make less noise if you run with your knees slightly bent.

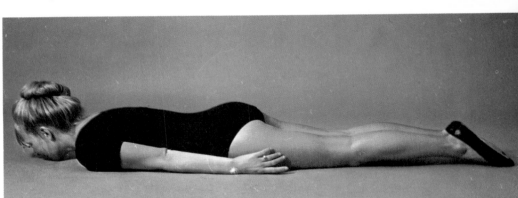

Right: Pull-ups. Lie down flat on your stomach, with your arms straight by your sides. Then raise your head and shoulders and both legs simultaneously from the floor, lifting as far as you can. Lower again. Do it twice.

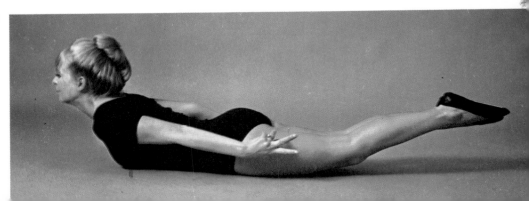

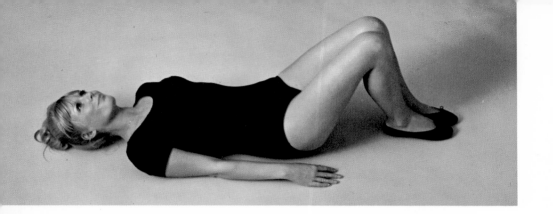

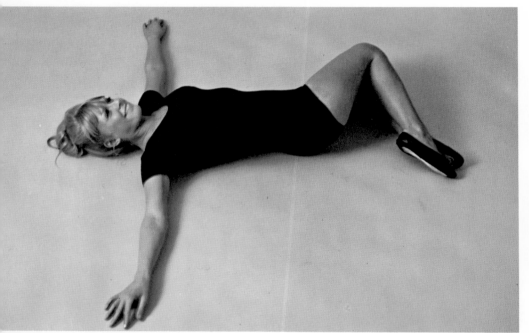

Left: Knee Swing. Lie on back with knees bent. Swing your knees over, first to the right, and then to the left, touching the floor on each side. Repeat eight times.

Right: Cossack Walk. Squat down with hands on hips, and walk six steps forward, staying in that position. Then walk six steps back again. It's easier to keep your balance if you bounce.

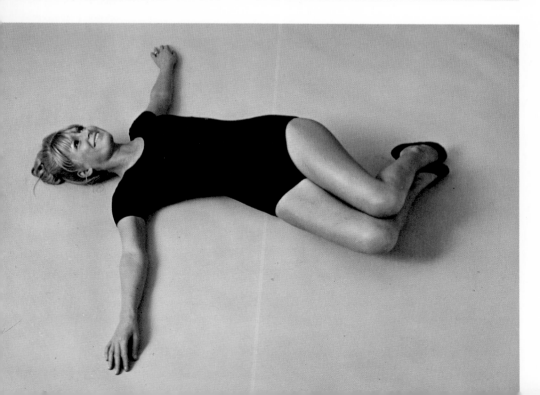

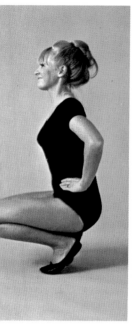
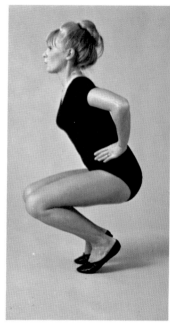
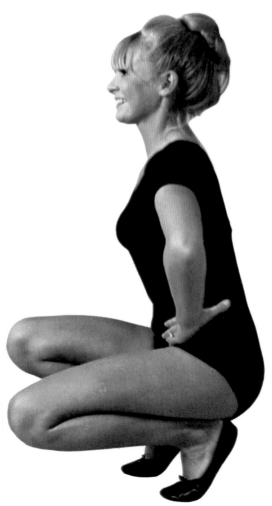

your back as straight as you can. Bending from the waist with your knees straight is bad for the back and can lead to needless aches and pains. Always try to push, rather than pull, heavy objects, and when stooping to lift something from the ground, bend right down, keeping your back straight and your knees well bent, rather than leaning over, arching your back and keeping your legs straight.

Even if you loathe the whole idea of routine exercising, or know, in your heart of hearts, that you will never manage to keep up a regular exercise program, there are lots of cunning little ways of fitting exercises into your daily routine without hardly even noticing it.

Anything that makes you stretch is good for you—even just stretching like a cat as you get out of bed. Bedmaking exercises lots of muscles. And so does dusting, provided you get right down on your knees and stretch your arms in a wide circle around you as you dust. Even taking a bath can be good exercise and tone up your circulation, if you give yourself a brisk allover scrub and a vigorous towelling afterward. After you have cleaned your teeth, you might even fit in a few knee-bending and stretching movements. Bend your knees while you support yourself with one hand on the washbasin, and then stretch up on tiptoe. The same exercise could be done at odd moments during the day, using the back of a chair or a door handle for support.

While you are doing the dishes, waiting for the bus, or sitting at your office desk, try a simple exercise for strengthening stomach muscles. Just pull in your stomach muscles, making sure you keep breathing naturally, and don't hold your breath. Hold for a count of six, relax, and then do the exercise again three or four times.

If you are on your feet a lot during the day, try to take a quick break now and again by literally putting your feet up. Lie on the floor and lean your legs against the nearest wall or chair for five minutes or so. And when you finally get to relax in front of the TV,

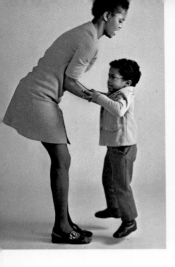
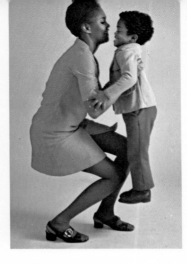

Above: your body can do a lot of work without overstrain if you use it right. To lift a child, bend the knees so that the legs take part of the weight. Below: the same principle of removing some of the load from your back applies when moving heavy furniture. Bend your knees, and it's a lot easier.

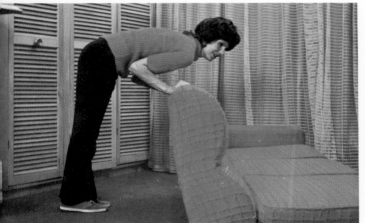

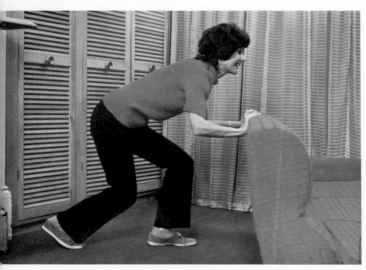

try this exercise during the breaks for commercials. Just sit well back in your chair, stretch up your arms and reach back as far as you can—as if you were having one long, elaborate, and refreshing yawn.

Exercise and diet are vital to good inner health, but they must be combined with adequate rest and relaxation. If your body and mind are tense, you will feel and look tired. But experts agree that you can do a lot to remove tension by learning how to breathe correctly. Most of us breathe too quickly and too shallowly. And when we are worried, we tend unconsciously to hold our breath as well as tensing our muscles.

One good breathing exercise that you can use to help you relax at odd moments during the day is to breathe in deeply through your nose and mouth, hold your breath for a count of three, and then breathe out very slowly, letting your head drop forward onto your chest as you empty your lungs.

Make it a general rule to slow your breathing and to breathe in and out deeply and regularly. And if you go to bed feeling tense and unable to sleep, try to breathe gently and slowly while you gradually relax each part of your body in turn. Start with your feet and then your legs, and so on gradually up the length of your body to your head. This sort of relaxation may take practice but it will ensure that you get a more refreshing night's sleep. For sleep is not necessarily restful by itself. Tense muscles can stay tense the whole night through, and that is one of the reasons why we often feel just as tired in the morning as we did the night before. But relaxed sleep is one of the best health and beauty treatments you can get.

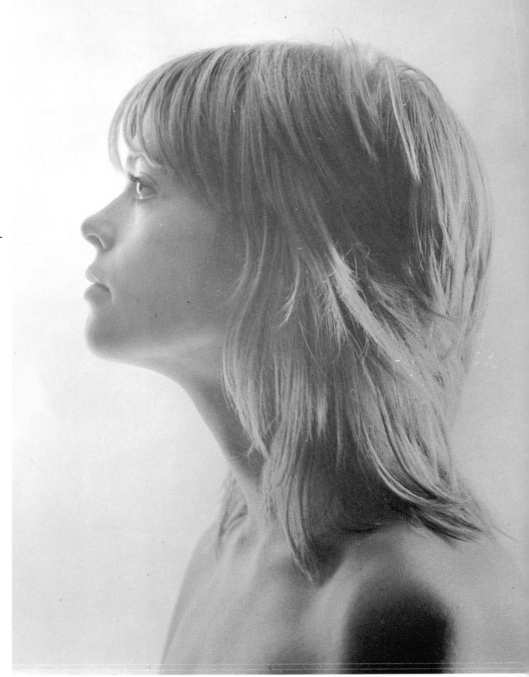

Right: a healthy body is always pleasant to look at. Powders and blushers can enhance your appearance, but they can't substitute for natural vitality.

Good inner health has plenty of beauty bonuses to offer. For the way you look depends far more on what is going on inside your body than on anything you do to the outside. And no amount of outer care can right the havoc caused by fatigue, tension, lack of exercise, or a faulty diet. So the best rule of all for looking good is to maintain your whole body in top condition.

Some women are, of course, born to be real beauties. But there is no evidence that this gift alone brings love or joy in life. Not every woman needs to be a beauty queen to have a rich, full life. Nevertheless, it is comforting to know that by being healthy, vigorous, fit—and, most of all, happy—every woman can *feel* beautiful. And when you feel that way, it shows.

111

An Ounce of Prevention
7

A women's magazine once featured an article entitled "Hypochondria is Good for You". What the writer really meant was that the healthy woman keeps an intelligent watch over her body to catch any abnormal condition before it gets out of hand and causes real trouble, not that she should spend her days worrying over slight aches and twinges or standing in front of her mirror painstakingly searching for signs of rare diseases. Such concern is in itself a form of ill health. Common sense, however, forces us to recognize that things can, and sometimes do, go wrong, despite the remarkable ability of your body to maintain itself, and regardless of the best of self-care programs. But before anything does go wrong, while you are in the best of health, it is wise to have your body machine checked up on a regular basis.

Good health adds so much sheer joy to life that it is a pity to miss even one day of healthy living. So why not make an ally of your doctor, who can evaluate your personal self-care program and detect any condition that might lead to ill health. Many, if not most, of the ills to which a woman's body is prone can be effectively dealt with if detected early enough. And that includes even the most serious.

For the sake of your life and health, let us take a look at the figures on three leading causes of needless and preventable early deaths among women. They are cancer of the breast, colon, and uterus. Just the word cancer alone sends a chill down the spine of most of us. We prefer not to know anything about it, even though knowledge saves mental anguish, prevents pain, and saves lives. For example, if breast cancer is detected and

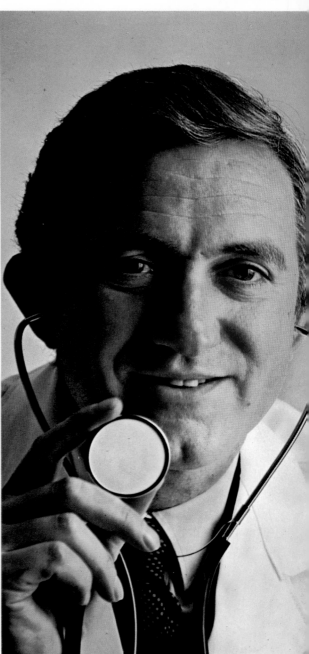

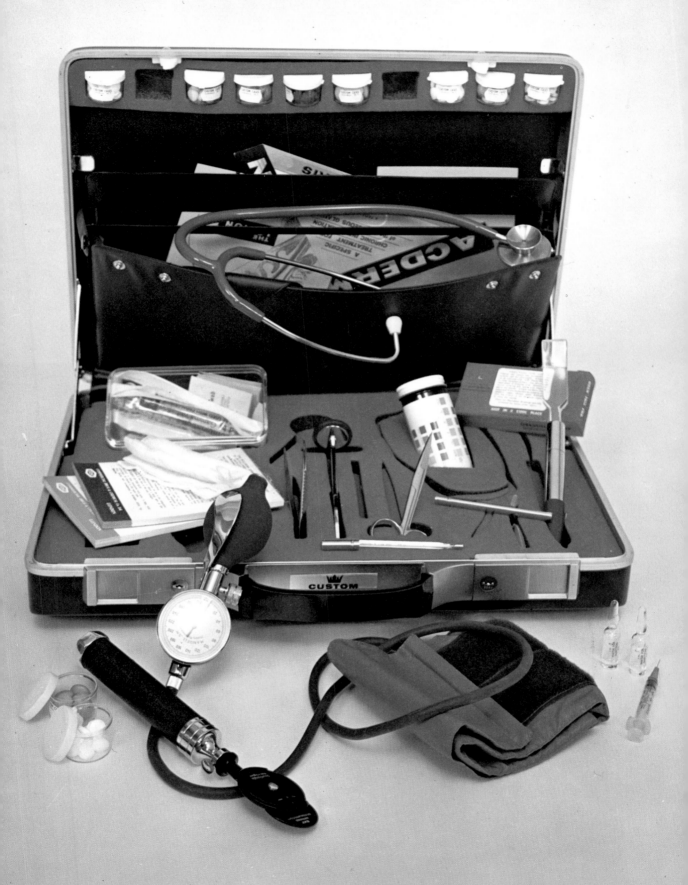

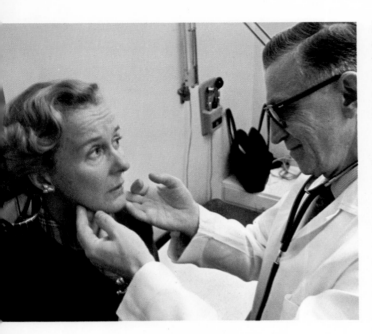

Above: if there is anything about your body that worries you, you should talk it over honestly with your doctor. No one can better relieve your worry.

treated while it is still restricted to the breast, the five-year survival rate (the percentage of women who are living five years later and deemed cured) is 85 per cent. Cancer of the colon, or large intestine, and rectum, is the number two cause of cancer death in both men and women. But most doctors believe that early detection and treatment of this form of cancer could result in a cure rate as high as 80 per cent. Cancer of the uterus, two-thirds of which occurs in the cervix (the part of the uterus that projects into the vagina) is diagnosed in 42,000 American women annually. But if it is caught in the very early stages, the patient has a 100 per cent chance of complete recovery.

Studies have indicated that 5 out of every 100 women stand a chance of developing cancer of the breast; 3 out of every 100 may develop cancer of the colon; between 2 and 3 may develop cancer of the cervix; and 2 may develop cancer of the body of the uterus. But doctors point out that women are luckier than men in that the parts of their body which are most prone to cancer, like the breasts and the uterus, are fairly easy to examine, and these types of cancer

lend themselves especially to early diagnosis, effective treatment and cure—provided a women goes for regular periodic checkups. For the only sure way of controlling and curing cancer is to detect it at the earliest possible moment.

In the past 50 years, medicine has made prodigious advances in the early detection of cancer and many other diseases. Improved diagnosis is the doctors' most powerful weapon in their efforts to keep you healthy. And the entire field of health care is now shifting increasingly toward the prevention and detection of disease before any obvious symptoms occur. All the statistics show that preventive health care is not only far more effective, but less costly. But payment aside, isn't it a lot easier and far pleasanter to accept the slight inconvenience of routine checks on your health than to risk the danger of disease? Or, if you want to look at it another way, simply consider that regluar health examinations are as much a part of your maintenance program as a good diet.

Specialists in preventive medicine recommend that every adult woman—from age 18 through the rest of her life—have a thorough professional medical checkup at least once a year. Now the sad truth is that it is not always easy to get a thorough medical exam. Many doctors are so busy treating disease that they may be reluctant to take valuable office time to examine the bodies of perfectly sound women. But this attitude is changing, and it is really up to you, for your health's sake, to see that you get a regular and thorough checkup. For that reason we have included the procedure followed by a leading American institution devoted to preventive medicine, so that you will know approximately what to expect during such a medical examination.

Typically, the examination begins with the taking of a detailed medical history. This includes quite a lot of probing questions, even some that may embarrass you. But only false shame would prevent your answering fully. The doctor must know exactly how you feel now, what medicines, if any, you

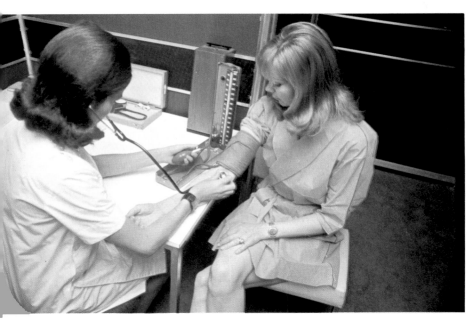

Your regular medical checkup will probably include some of these tests in which sophisticated machines are used. They often reveal abnormalities of which you may not have had any symptoms at all.

Left: checking of blood pressure is a routine. Middle: examining your eyes for unsuspected blind spots. This is a problem to which heavy smokers are susceptible. Below left: a test given to check the range of sounds heard properly. Below right: testing the volume of air your lungs take in with each breath.

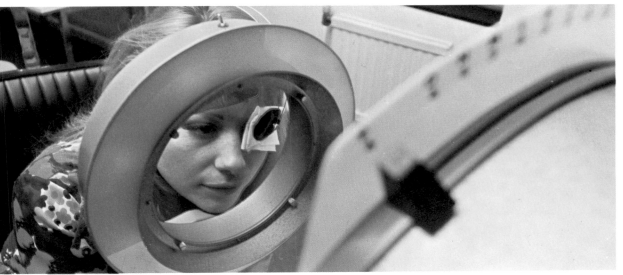

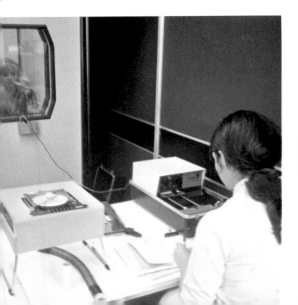

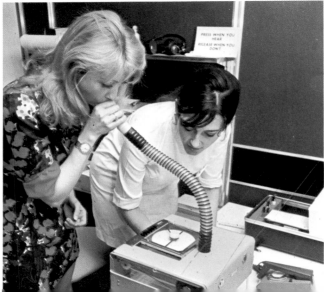

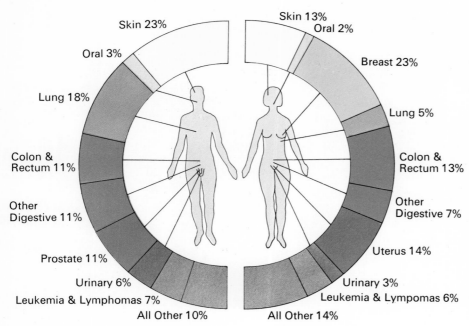

Skin 23%
Oral 3%
Lung 18%
Colon & Rectum 11%
Other Digestive 11%
Prostate 11%
Urinary 6%
Leukemia & Lymphomas 7%
All Other 10%

Skin 13%
Oral 2%
Breast 23%
Lung 5%
Colon & Rectum 13%
Other Digestive 7%
Uterus 14%
Urinary 3%
Leukemia & Lympomas 6%
All Other 14%

Left. the parts of the body most susceptible to cancer differ in men and women. This chart shows the incidence of cancer for both of the sexes.

Right: you are the person who can do the most to keep your body functioning as it should. Your own program of maintenance—shown by blue dots—and regular checkups—shown by red dots—are the best ways of guaranteeing a healthy body for yourself. Also, keep alert for the six warning symptoms listed by the American Cancer Association, and go to your doctor at once if you notice any.

are taking, and what has happened to you in the past. The doctor will also want to know whether any of your blood relatives have suffered from diabetes, allergy, or high blood pressure, so that he can be on the alert for any early signs of these diseases.

The actual physical examination might begin with an overall inspection of your body to detect any superficial signs of disease or other conditions. Doctors can learn a great deal from skin color and texture, any unusual lumps or swellings and from gently prodding and probing a number of strategic locations on your body. The examination will probably include your scalp, eyes, ears, nose, throat, and the rest of your body, right down to your feet. A stethoscope will be used to listen to the sounds made by your heart and lungs as air goes in and out. This examination plus your own comments and complaints, if any, will determine to a large extent what other tests and examinations should be performed.

Depending on your doctor, he may feel that certain other tests are necessary. These may include x-rays, from both front and side, to detect any abnormalities or early signs of disease in the chest cavity; blood counts; analysis of a urine sample; and possibly an

1. Any sore that doesn't heal quickly, especially around the mouth or on the vulva.
2. Any persistent hoarseness or cough, or difficulty in swallowing.
3. Any painless lump, especially in the breasts, lips, tongue, or soft tissues.
4. Any persistent indigestion or unexplained loss in your weight.
5. Any unexplained change in normal bowel habits.
6. Any unusual bleeding or discharge from any natural body opening, especially the vagina.

electrocardiogram—a recording of the electrical impulses from the heart. Many women, particularly younger ones, are surprised at this examination because they do not normally think of themselves as potential heart disease victims. Unfortunately, women in their late teens and early twenties do sometimes have heart abnormalities. Furthermore, the electrocardiagram reveals more about you than just the condition of your heart. It can also indicate abnormalities in the chemical balance of the blood or in the autonomic nervous system which serves the heart. For this reason, some doctors do include this test in their annual checkups of even young women.

X-rays of your abdomen are not called for in a regular annual checkup unless other clues make your doctor think them necessary.

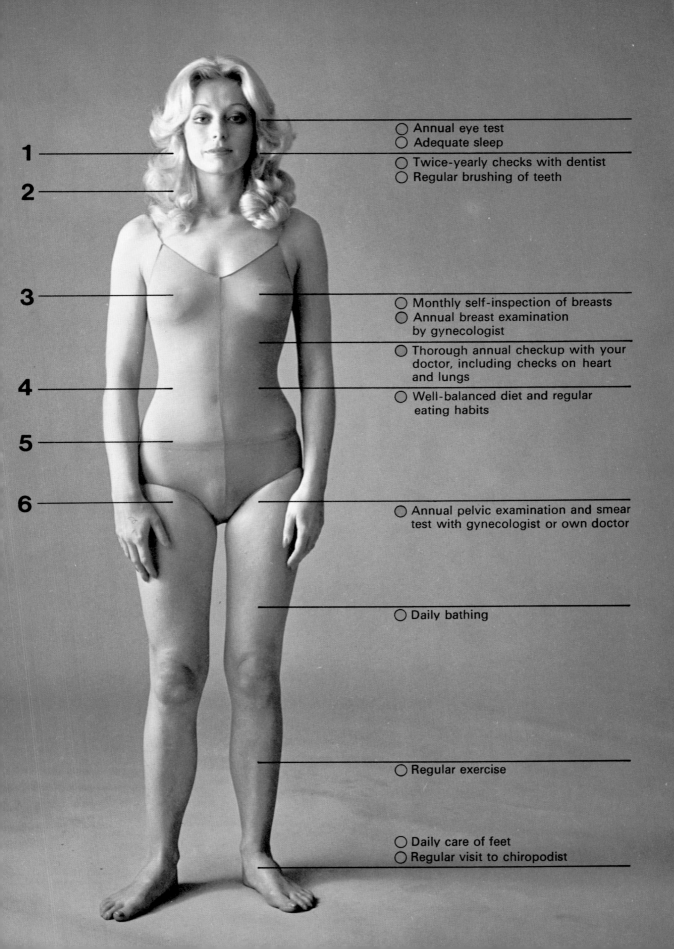

1

2

3

4

5

6

○ Annual eye test
○ Adequate sleep
○ Twice-yearly checks with dentist
○ Regular brushing of teeth

○ Monthly self-inspection of breasts
○ Annual breast examination
   by gynecologist
○ Thorough annual checkup with your
   doctor, including checks on heart
   and lungs
○ Well-balanced diet and regular
   eating habits

○ Annual pelvic examination and smear
   test with gynecologist or own doctor

○ Daily bathing

○ Regular exercise

○ Daily care of feet
○ Regular visit to chiropodist

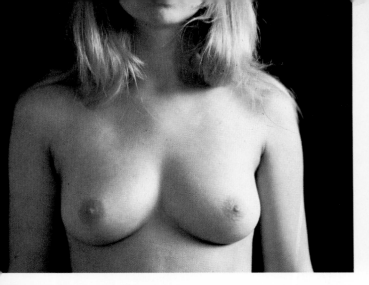

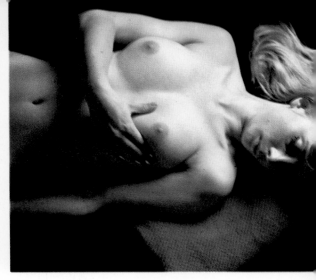

2 Now lie down and put a folded towel under your left shoulder. Holding your fingers together and using the fingertips only, feel the lower outer quarter of your breast. Be gentle but firm, and keep your left arm down.

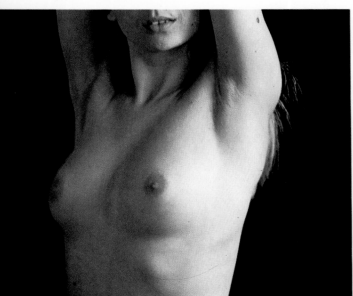

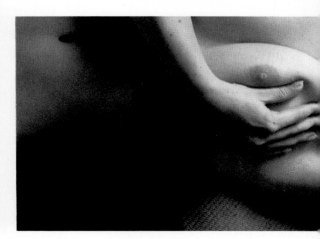

1 Sitting in front of your mirror, look for any change in shape or puckering of the skin. First check with your arms hanging loosely at your sides. Then check with your arms raised, while you turn from side to side.

Above: self-examination for breast tumors is not hard, doesn't take long, and—say the doctors—is essential for women of all ages. The checkup, as described step by step, should be done each month.

Similarly, the inspection of the interior of the rectum and colon may not be required more than once every two or three years.

In addition to following up any clues discovered in your medical history or in the initial examination, the doctor will probably measure your height and weight, and study

3 In the same position, examine the upper outer quarter of your breast. Begin close to the nipple, where you left off with the inner quarter, and move your fingers steadily and gently toward the armpit.

the pattern of fat distribution on your body. Additional blood tests may be ordered to determine the amount and kinds of fat in your blood stream. Finally, if any kind of deteriorating condition is detected, the doctor will prescribe an appropriate treatment to arrest it. This may involve nothing more than a change in routine, simple rest, or medication. In some cases, of course, an operation may be called for to put things in the proper working order.

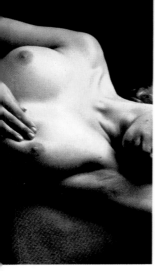
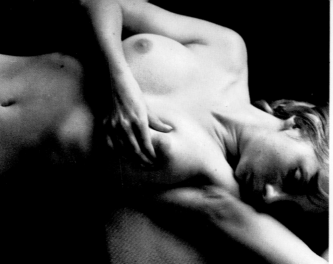
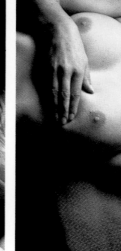

Then put your left hand under your head. In that position, check the lower inner quarter, starting just under the nipple.

4 Still lying down, with your arm behind your head, check the upper inner quarter. Press gently to feel any lump or slight thickening. Work from the outer edge toward the nipple, and then press gently around the nipple with your fingertips. (You will soon learn the characteristic shape and features of your own breast, and recognise any changes).

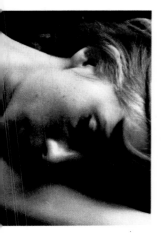
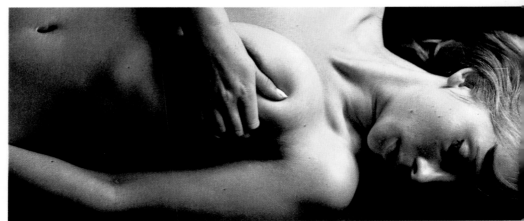

5 Then put your arm back down by your side, and check the upper outer quarter again. This time, feel directly under the armpit for any lumps or thickening. Then put the folded towel under your right shoulder, and use your left hand to check the right breast just as you did the other breast. Be sure to see your doctor about anything unusual.

This annual routine checkup, however, does not end your responsibility. At least once a year—twice, if possible—you should visit your gynecologist (the medical specialist devoted to maintaining the health of your reproductive system). Or if you are unable to find a gynecologist in your area, ask your doctor for an annual pelvic examination. This will include a careful inspection of your entire pelvic area, and a Pap smear. This vital smear test (named for Dr. George

Papanicolaou who invented it) is used to detect cancer of the cervix, and every woman should make sure she has such a test at least once a year. In fact, many specialists recommend it be made twice a year. A Pap smear consists of a microscopic examination of cells cast off by the cervix that are collected from the vagina. Collection of the cells in a doctor's office is fast and completely painless. The Pap test can detect abnormal changes in tissue five to ten years before symptoms of

119

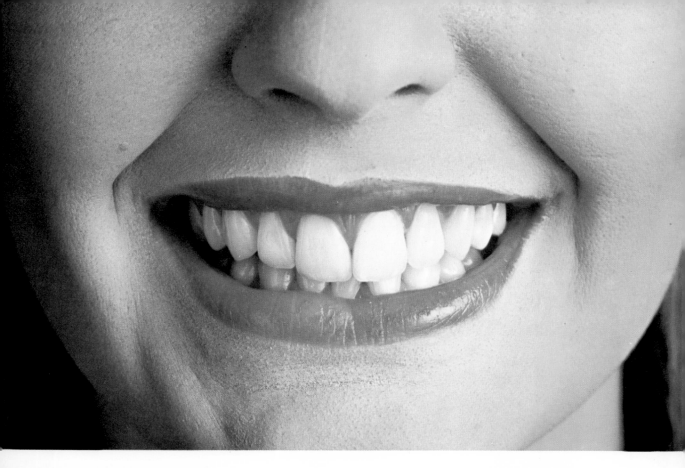

Above: your smile is your greeting to the world, and the sparkle of healthy teeth belongs with it.

cancer begin to appear. Only by Pap smears and by regular pelvic examinations, doctors say, will cervical cancer be eliminated as a major cause of women's deaths.

The gynecologist will also perform a breast examination to detect any suspicious lumps. It is important to remember, however, that, although breast tumors and cysts are quite common, the majority of them are benign—that is, they are not cancerous. If a lump is discovered, the doctor may order it to be surgically removed to determine whether it is benign. This requires a very small incision that often leaves no scar whatever afterwards. Some women have a tendency to develop benign breast tumors and may have four or five removed in the course of their lifetime without any permanent damaging effects either to their overall health or to their breasts.

Even though benign tumors are far more common than malignant ones, it is vital to have any lump in the breast evaluated as quickly as possible. That is the only way to set your mind at rest, or, on the chance that it may be cancer, the way to be cured, and enjoy a healthy, happy life.

Because the detection of breast tumors is so important, gynecologists recommend monthly self-inspections. Your own breast examination should follow the method shown on page 118-119, and should be done within a day or two after your period is over. This vital self-inspection should continue for the rest of your life even after your menopause.

In addition to this regular inspection of her breasts, a woman can also help herself to escape serious disease just by being alert to any unusual changes in the functioning of her body. See page 116 for a list of symptoms considered by the American Cancer Association to call for immediate consultation with a doctor.

Of course, these symptoms may be due to many causes apart from cancer. But doctors

120

agree that if all women followed the American Cancer Association's advice, there would be a tremendous increase in the rate of cancer cure. So remember that misplaced fear should never prevent you from going to a doctor. Early diagnosis means that effective treatment can be given, and the chances of complete cure are very high.

An ounce of prevention is always better than a pound of cure. And prevention doesn't just mean detecting illness early, but also making sure that you keep every part of your body in the very best of health. Among other things, this involves a regular, twice-yearly visit to your dentist.

Your dentist will not only inspect your teeth for the beginnings of tooth decay or gum disease, but will also clean them to remove a very hard substance called *tartar* that forms on them. Tartar can cause dangerous irritations and gum disease, and cannot be entirely removed by the toothbrush. Interestingly, after the age of 25, most people lose teeth not because of tooth decay, but because of gum disease and a deterioration of the bone that hold the teeth in place. This is completely avoidable with proper dental care.

You should take care of your teeth above all by brushing them regularly. Toothbrushing performs two important functions. First, it removes tiny particles of food that stick to teeth and between them. If left in the mouth, food particles are acted on by saliva to form powerful acids that are capable of attacking the tooth enamel that protects teeth—and cavities result. Secondly, toothbrushing sharply reduces the accumulation of tartar that must be removed by the dentist. Once dry, the tartar is very hard and not affected by the toothbrush, but in the first 24 hours after its deposition, it is softer and can be brushed away.

Teeth should be brushed at least twice a day, night and morning, or *after* meals. Brushing at night before going to bed is particularly important, because while you are asleep, the supply of saliva slows down and food debris has no chance of being

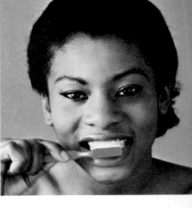

Brushing your teeth not only helps the teeth themselves—by removing food particles that might cause decay—but also helps the gums—by giving them stimulation.

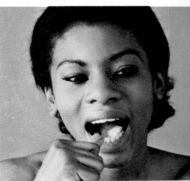

Always brush your teeth with an up-and-down movement. The use of a sideways movement can wear down the surface.

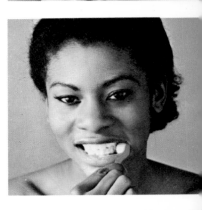

Be sure to brush the back as well as the front, reaching well back to do the molars deep inside the mouth.

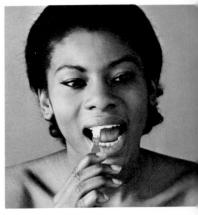

Be sure to replace a wornout toothbrush immediately. Bristles that stick out not only can hurt your gums, but also fail to clean thoroughly.

washed away from between the teeth.

Teeth should be cleaned by brushing gently but firmly from the gums toward the tips (see illustration on page 121). Sideways brushing can damage teeth and gums and will not remove food particles efficiently. You can use a circular movement, but be careful not to push the gums back from the teeth, as this may expose the sensitive base of the teeth which is more easily attacked by decay. Remember, too, to include the gums in your toothbrushing routine. Careful brushing will massage the gums and help prevent gum disease.

Your toothbrush should not be too hard, and brushing should not be too vigorous, as this may make the gums bleed. Electric toothbrushes can help by massaging the gums, but otherwise have no particular advantage over ordinary toothbrushes except perhaps for encouraging children to brush their teeth by making it more fun.

Toothpaste, of course, helps you to brush and puts a pleasant taste in your mouth. Some women also like to finish off with a mouthwash to give them a really fresh-tasting mouth and sweet-smelling breath. Mouth deodorants, however, are a more controversial subject. They act by disguising unpleasant tastes or bad breath, and are not effective for everyone. When bad breath is a persistent problem, and not just the result of eating pungent foods (like onions, garlic, or alcohol), or of smoking, the only solution is to seek the root of the trouble and get it attended to. Bad breath is often due to decaying food particles lodged in a tooth cavity or trapped under flaps of skin in the

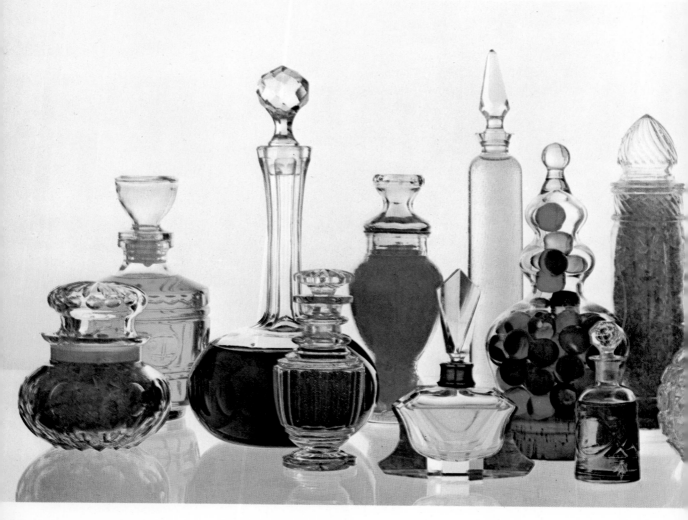

gums, and a dentist can soon take care of the problem. Alternatively, bad breath may be the result of an upset stomach, and, if it persists, it is best to consult a doctor.

A woman's life is meant to be lived fully. Part of the fullness is seeing what goes on in the world about you. Your yearly health maintenance program is not complete unless it includes a visit to an eye doctor. If you need corrective lenses, you will find that the proper prescription will help relieve headaches and tension. And glasses have a lasting cosmetic effect. They will eliminate the hard-to-erase wrinkles and crows' feet that come from squinting.

Your eye doctor may also include a test for glaucoma in his checkup. Glaucoma is a condition in which fluid pressure in the eyeball causes destruction of the retina—the part of the eye that receives the light rays. This is the commonest cause of blindness among adults in the Western world, and is most often found after age 35 to 40. But glaucoma is another of those diseases that can be successfully and easily treated if discovered in time.

You can also do a lot yourself to keep your eyes clear and sparkling. First of all, you should make sure you get an adequate amount of sleep and eat a well-balanced diet. Try also to rest your eyes during the day by this simple exercise: look up as far as you can and then down as far as you can; look to the

Relaxing in a warm bath after a long day can give a special delight to a woman, in addition to bringing a fresh feeling of cleanliness. There is something luxurious about a slow, lazy bath—especially if the water is scented and softened with oils or salts.

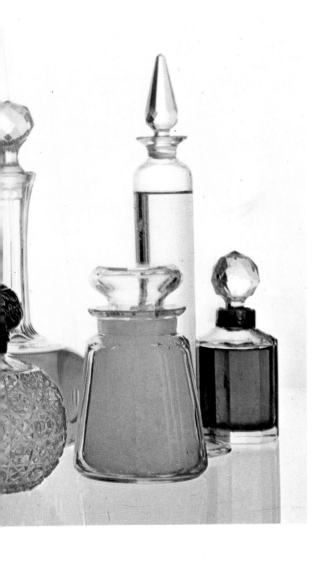

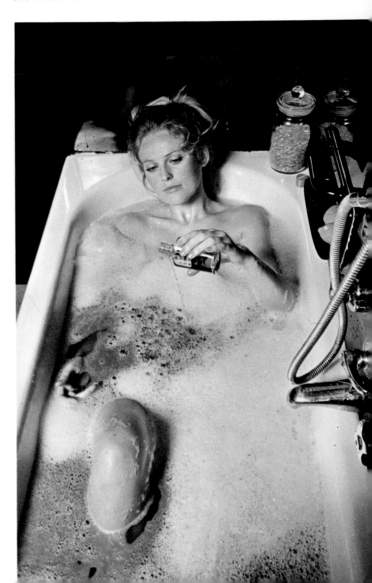

Clean and fresh after your bath, you are probably ready to use some of the beauty products that give one more touch to your care of your body. Many women like nail polish to brighten finger or toenails; most women consider deodorants essential.

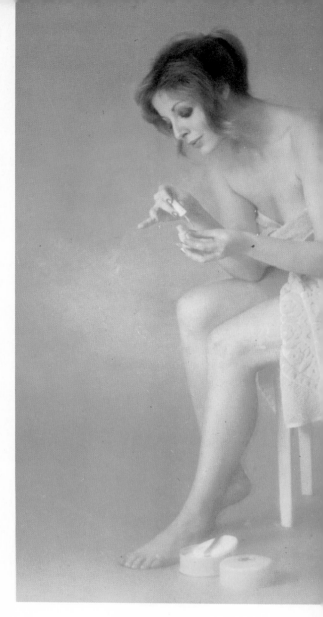

left and then to the right until you can see as far as possible out of the corner of your eyes; then roll your eyes round and blink a few times. If you do a lot of close work, rest your eyes as frequently as possible by looking up and as far into the distance as you can.

Be careful to keep make-up out of your eyes and always clean off eye make-up gently but thoroughly at night. Eye drops or lotions can be soothing, and some eye drops will make eyes look brighter by constricting the tiny blood vessels that can redden them. Eye compresses or cotton soaked in eye lotion can also refresh tired eyes. Last but not least, try to avoid frowning, which not only wrinkles the forehead but also creases the sensitive skin around the eyes. And if you find that you are frowning a lot, it is almost certainly time to see your eye doctor for a test.

One other expert whose help you may need in your health maintenance program is the chiropodist. Some experts believe that we should visit a chiropodist as often as we go to the dentist. For, they point out, our feet have a great deal to bear—especially if we are plumper than we should be.

To strengthen the muscles in your feet, chiropodists recommend standing barefoot, or in stockinged feet, and scratching the floor with your toes, then stretching out your feet and turning the toes up. Arches can also be strengthened simply by walking around the house on tiptoe for a couple of minutes during the day.

Caring for your feet is, of course, most easily done as part of your regular bathtime routine. And no woman needs to be told that hygiene—or, to put it plainly, keeping clean—is one of the most important aspects of staying healthy, as well as the basis of good grooming. But how often should a woman bathe? At least every two days, say doctors—and preferably once a day. Sur-

prisingly, some doctors maintain that women do not normally need to use soap, since plain water is enough to wash away all bacteria and most accumulated dirt. But most women would probably find dirt pretty hard to get rid of without soap, and doctors agree that, for practical purposes, it is best to use a gentle soap and plenty of warm water, either in a tub or shower. Antiseptic soaps, however, are not necessary —unless prescribed by a doctor for a skin complaint—and may even be harmful, particularly in the sensitive vulva area (see Chapter 1). Antiseptics may not only kill harmful bacteria but also the useful bacteria

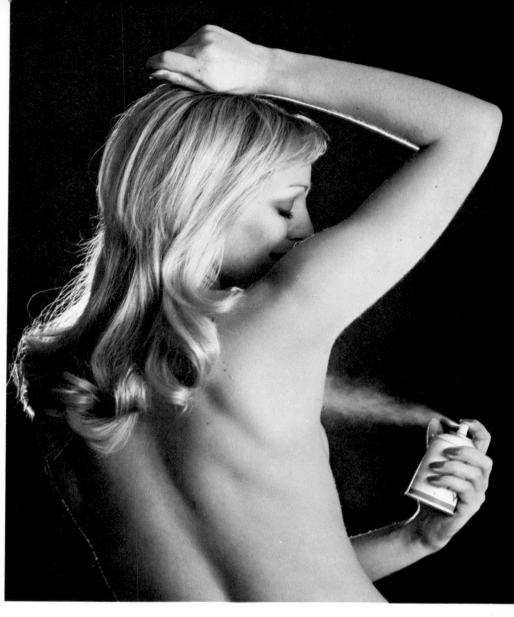

that protect skin from infection. Careful intimate hygiene is a must, but should be carried out with the mildest of soaps and warm water. Some women find that even gentle soaps irritate the sensitive areas around the vagina, and, in this case, it is best to use only plain water, although soap should be used to help cleanse the pubic hairs thoroughly. Alternatively, doctors can recommend a special type of soap.

No deodorant or antiperspirant can take the place of regular washing or of keeping your clothes fresh and clean. Deodorants act by masking odors, usually with a perfume of their own, and antiperspirants check a certain amount of perspiration. Often the two are combined in a single product. Antiperspirants usually work by plugging the pores to prevent the normal flow of secretions. Fortunately, most of them are unable to prevent perspiration entirely. When they do, skin problems often occur. A new kind of antiperspirant that employs a kind of drug that acts directly on the nerves and the sweat glands they serve may be even more harmful. By blocking the nerve impulses that cause the glands to secrete, these antiperspirants literally stop the secretions. And any such tampering with the natural body processes can obviously be exceedingly dangerous. Both doctors and various government health officials and agencies are becoming increasingly concerned about the harm such antiperspirants cause, and, in a growing number of cases, have succeeded in legally removing them from the marketplace.

If you have a problem of excessive perspiration, it may be the result of nervousness and worry that can overactivate the sweat glands. In this case, worrying will only increase the problem, so the best course of action is to enlist the help of your doctor.

Another major offender in the field of feminine hygiene is the vaginal deodorant. Advertisements for these products often succeed in making a woman feel less confident and less feminine if she does not use an intimate deodorant. In fact, as most doctors point out, the average woman who bathes every day has no need whatsoever to use a vaginal deodorant. The vagina, say gynecologists, is equipped by Nature to keep itself clean, and, although the vaginal area (like the penis) may have a natural faint odor, this is quite undetectable to other people, unless a woman has skipped or skimped her bathing.

Apart from scrupulous washing, especially during her periods, a woman should also change her underwear every day without fail. Interestingly enough, the wearing of pants by women is a relatively recent innovation. When pants were introduced from the harems of the East about 100 years ago, women thought them quite indecent— possibly because the first Westerners to adopt them were French prostitutes. Now, of course, it is generally considered indecent not to wear pants. But unfortunately we have mostly chosen fairly close-fitting pants and tights, which shut in an area of the body that is normally warm and moist and thus more susceptible to chafing and infection. Some doctors talk regretfully of the pre-panty era, when air had a chance of reaching that part of the body and keeping it as healthy as any other part. They do not, however, suggest you strike a blow for

feminine health by burning your pants— just that you choose a kind that allow a certain amount of air to circulate around the skin, and that you change your undies daily. They also recommend absorbent material in preference to nylon.

On another aspect of feminine hygiene, doctors are not so firmly agreed. This is the question of douching. Many gynecologists consider douching unnecessary because of the vagina's ability to cleanse itself by its special secretion. An ordinary tub bath, they say, will insure the removal of any odor. These gynecologists also warn that douching tends to wash away too much of the protective substances in the vagina and may harm delicate tissues there. Other doctors disagree. They think that the vagina may sometimes fail to do an adequate self-cleaning job and therefore needs the occasional help of a douche. At this point, the answer to the question must come from the individual woman. If she finds that ordinary careful daily washing is satisfactory, then nothing more is required. If she is not satisfied, she might try a gentle douche as often as she feels is needed—perhaps once a week or every two weeks.

All in all, the maintenance required to keep your body in the peak of condition is relatively minimal, a few hours each year, less probably by many times than you spend watching television or at the cinema or theater. A woman must be vigilant about detecting any signs of deterioration in her health and quick to react in correcting the situation. And she must be consistent in regularly obtaining professional help to monitor the functioning of her body and correct minor problems as they occur. This simple application of a mere ounce of prevention can virtually guarantee that you will add happy, healthful, and vital life to your years—as well as years to your life.

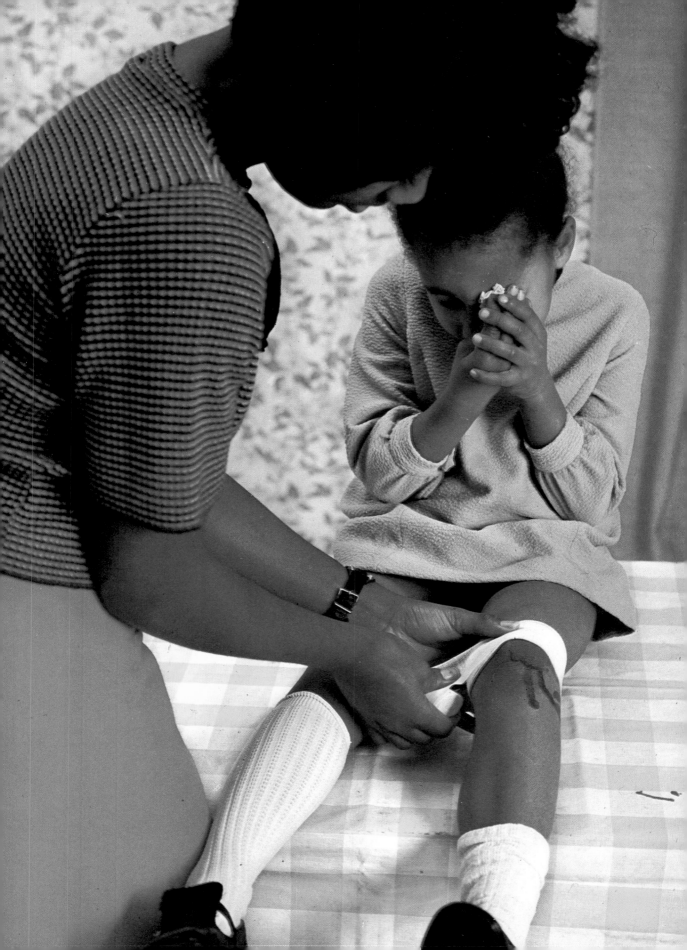

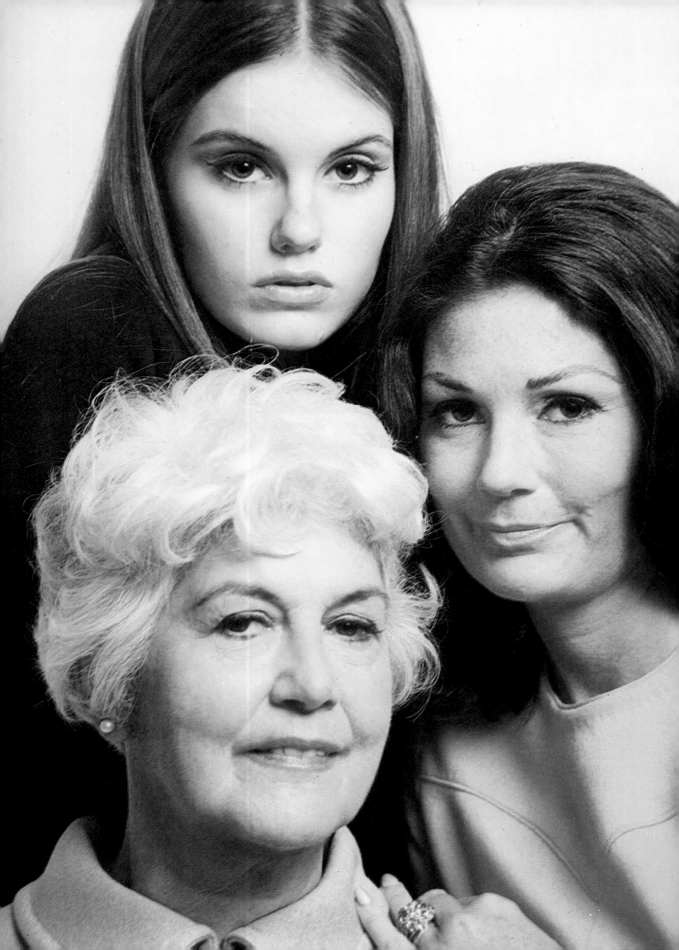

Questions & Answers

Is there any way of telling when I will have my menopause? Is it normal for one breast to be larger than the other? How will a hysterectomy affect my sex life? Can hormone pills cause cancer? How many eggs does a woman have in her ovaries? Do women age faster than men?

In the following pages you will find the answers to these and many other questions of particular interest to women of all ages. Topics discussed include sleeping, dreaming, and the best ways of dealing with insomnia; the facts about the "change of life," what it means, what effects it may have, and how to deal with them; the years that come after and the exciting prospects for prolonging active life; the causes and cures of some of the disorders that worry women most; when and why an operation may be needed and what difference it will make to your life; and finally, some fascinating and little-known facts about a woman's body.

Here are the answers to some of the questions most often raised about the whys and wherefores of being a woman, and practical advice on how to handle some of the upsets that can so often cause needless anxiety and concern. All of us have to face health problems of one kind or another at some time in our lives. But by dispelling many common fears about the special health problems faced by women, this information is designed to guide you safely through life's difficult days and to help you feel happy and confident about your health.

This information is not intended to replace the advice of a doctor, for you should always seek medical advice on any problem that affects your health. On the contrary, it is meant to supplement the information he may give you, to answer some of the questions you may hestitate, or forget, to ask him, and, above all, to help you know more about yourself. For knowing about our bodies and understanding the problems that may beset them from time to time is the most important step toward achieving long and lasting good health.

Left: daughter, mother, and grandmother—all in the glow of good health, and all looking beautiful for it. In today's world it is easy to get the information we need in order to protect and maintain our bodies for a vigorous and happy life at every age.

Sleep

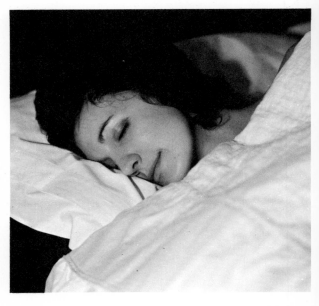

Why do we need to sleep?

Surprisingly enough, no one really knows, for research into sleep is relatively new. But the first full-scale investigation of sleep, held only 20 years ago, did reveal some vital facts about the way we sleep. Researchers discovered that there are two distinct kinds of sleep—dreaming and non-dreaming—that follow a definite pattern every night. As you go to sleep, you sink by stages into a non-dreaming sleep. But an hour or so later, you slip back to the lesser stages of unconsciousness that you began with. And your eyes start to flicker about beneath your eyelids as if you were watching a movie. You have started to dream. And throughout the night this dreaming sleep will alternate regularly with periods of dreamless sleep.

While you sleep, your heart beats less fast and your breathing slows down. Your temperature and blood pressure drop, and your kidneys secrete far less urine. Your hands grow colder and your feet warmer. Your sweat glands are more active, and you actually lose several ounces in weight while asleep. During the night, you turn over about 40 times, often in response to the action of your dreams.

So sleep brings about considerable changes in your body functioning. But the reason why the body needs to "switch off" in this way for about one-third of each day remains a mystery. Some experts suggest that sleep helps to repair and renew our brain and body tissues. Non-dreaming sleep works on the body, they say, and dreaming sleep on the brain. Others hold the view that sleep gives our brain a chance to sort out and file away the mass of information that bombards it during the day. Dreams, they suggest, are just glimpses of this "tidying-up" process. Another theory is that the mind needs sleep and dreams as an escape from the frustrations of reality. But whatever the reasons for sleep, we cannot possibly do without it. Ten days is as long as an average person can manage to stay awake. And by the third day without sleep, most people begin to suffer from visual illusions, start laughing for no apparent reason, and easily become aggressive. As time wears on, the sleepless person begins to have regular hallucinations. And no matter how hard they struggle to stay awake, they tend to fall into short dozes of a few seconds' duration—so overwhelming is the body's mysterious need for sleep.

How much sleep do you need?

Sleep needs vary widely from one person to another. Some people find that as little as three or four hours' sleep is enough. Others train themselves to take short naps during the day and so need less sleep at night. Everybody has his own unique sleep pattern. But the majority of people between the ages of 30 and 80 sleep, on average, about $7\frac{1}{2}$ hours a night. Younger people need more sleep—maybe as much as 10 or 12 hours in their teens—and older people sleep less—around 5 hours. Babies sleep most, averaging about 16 hours a day. However, as every mother knows, even babies have their own individual sleep habits. Some may sleep, on and off, for as many as 23 hours out of 24; others for 13 hours or less. Girls often sleep more soundly than boys, but there is no evidence to suggest that women need more or less sleep than men. Nor is there any evidence to back up the idea that sleeping early at night does you more good than over-sleeping in the morning—it's the number of hours that count. And although too little sleep hampers health and efficiency, there doesn't seem to be any advantage in having extra sleep. Experiments during which people were allowed to sleep two hours more than usual have shown that they were actually less efficient after their longer sleep.

What causes insomnia, and how can it be cured?

True insomnia—the inability to sleep at all—is very rare indeed. But many people suffer from difficulties in getting to sleep, restless and inadequate sleep, or early waking. And, as anyone who has ever suffered from sleeplessness knows, there's nothing worse than tossing and turning in a state of wakefulness while the rest of the world is asleep. Sleeplessness may be due to many causes, including discomfort from physical illness, preoccupation with the worries of the day, late-night snacks, or just the off-putting effect of a strange bed, unaccustomed surroundings, or a noisy, airless, or chilly bedroom. Quarrels—often arising from tiredness—may prevent sleep. And an exciting TV program just before bedtime can make sleep difficult. Coffee drunk late in the evening will stimulate the brain. And cigarettes, alcohol, or even an empty stomach are just as bad. Difficulty in sleeping often occurs during pregnancy and menopause. But far and away the commonest causes of sleeplessness are depression and anxiety. Depression is a frequent cause of waking in the middle of the night or very early in the morning. Anxiety, on the other hand, is characterized by difficulty in getting to sleep.

For, as we begin to fall asleep, our reason and sense of proportion are quickly lost. And as reason weakens, imagination takes a stronger hold, making even minor worries assume alarming proportions. Many mothers cannot sleep until their teenage children are safely home and in bed. Other women find that sleep eludes them as they worry over the affairs of the previous day or the problems of the next. They may then start to worry over not being able to sleep, and build up a vicious circle of anxiety and sleeplessness.

No matter what the cause of poor sleep, it is important to seek the advice of a doctor. He may prescribe sleeping pills, which, used over a short period of time, can help reaccustom your body and mind to the sleeping habit until you can manage to sleep without them. But the type of drug he prescribes—if any—will depend on his assessment of your sleep problem. That's why it is so important not to borrow sleeping pills—what is all right for one person may be all wrong for another.

Other methods of curing sleeplessness vary from hypnosis and yoga to electronic sleep machines. Hypnosis works by helping a person learn how to suggest to himself that he will sleep—and wake—at given times. But it doesn't work for everybody. Yoga can help make sleep easier by teaching you how to relax. Sleep machines play a kind of electronic lullaby to the brain. But they involve wearing electrodes on the scalp—and must be used under medical supervision. The best way to tackle occasional sleep problems is to make sure you get enough fresh air and exercise, and to do your best to keep the day's aggravations from dragging on into the evening. Before going to bed, take time over some relaxing activity that you enjoy—a leisurely beauty routine, a warm bath, some light reading or music. A warm drink can also help. Make sure your bed is as cosy and inviting as possible, and that your bedroom is well-aired but not too cold. And, once in bed, don't start worrying about not getting to sleep—losing sleep will do you less harm than worrying about it. Breathe deeply and regularly, relax your muscles, and let your mind wander over pleasant things that calm and comfort you until sleep comes.

How long do dreams usually last, and how many dreams can you have in one night?

Most people spend about 2 hours a night dreaming. A baby dreams for about half of its sleep time—premature babies even more—and this gradually lessens as a child grows up.

Dreaming occurs about five times during the night, at intervals of 1 to 1½ hours. Dreaming sleep may last for periods of 10 to 30 minutes during the first part of the night, and for as long as an hour toward the end of the night. But recent research has shown that, even during non-dreaming sleep, the mind is never totally blank.

I never dream. Is this abnormal?

In fact, you do dream. Everybody dreams. Even people who are blind from birth dream as vividly as a sighted person, although their dreams usually involve hearing and feeling instead of visual images. But most of our dreams are forgotten, and some people just don't remember their dreams at all. Remembering dreams depends largely on when you wake up. Nearly everyone can recall a dream if they are waked during the rapid eye movements that normally denote dreaming sleep. But few people will remember dreams if waked even 10 minutes after these eye movements stop. Dreams are so important to humans that, if they are prevented from dreaming during experiments, they remain tense and irritable all the next day—even if they had a full seven or eight hours' sleep. And as soon as they can get an uninterrupted period of sleep, they spend double the usual time dreaming. This need to dream may also explain why people deprived of sleep for long periods suffer from hallucinations. These hallucinations tend to occur at the same frequency as dreams do in sleep—as if the brain were trying to follow the normal sleep pattern.

Do animals dream?

Most pet owners have noticed times when their sleeping dog or cat seems to be in hot pursuit of some imaginary quarry. This is not just fancy, for all seeing animals dream. And their need to dream is just as great as ours. A sleep experiment proved, for example that cats will die within three weeks if they are deprived of dreaming. And some animals seem to need more dream time than others. Cats are avid dreamers, often spending more than half their sleep time dreaming. But sheep dream for only two per cent of their sleep time. Does a cat have more on its mind than a sheep? No one knows.

Why do some people snore? And is there a cure?

Persistent snoring is often due to the sleeping person's position in bed. Snorers tend to lie on their backs with their mouths open, and may be temporarily cured by turning—or being pushed!—onto their sides. Occasionally, snoring is due to swellings in the lining of the nose, which should receive medical treatment. Other causes may be a loss of tone in palate muscles—more likely in an older person—or difficulty in closing the mouth. Children rarely snore, but, if they do, swollen tonsils or adenoids may be at the root of the trouble, and a doctor should be consulted. Temporary snoring is often due to a cold or any infection that blocks the nose. Sometimes snoring started during a cold may just become a habit. Snoring, which affects both sexes equally, has also been put down to smoking, overweight, fatigue, overwork—or a deformed nose. Embarrassing and inelegant though it may be, snoring is quite harmless to the snorer. And—as the partners of snorers know only too well—it doesn't disturb the snorer's sleep in the slightest. Countless suggested remedies for snoring include strapping a tennis ball or a hairbrush to the small of the back to prevent the sleeper from lying flat, using extra pillows to prop up the head, keeping his mouth closed with a peg—or investing in a pair of ear plugs.

The Change of Life

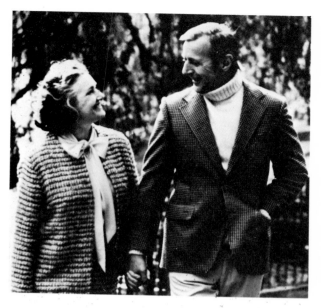

What is the "change of life" and why does it happen?

The "change of life," or menopause, is the time in a woman's life when her ovaries stop releasing eggs and her periods cease. But this is no sudden and isolated event. And the term "change of life" is usually applied to the whole series of physical and psychological changes that occur as a woman's childbearing capacity tapers off. The sequence of events begins—for some reason as yet unknown—when the pituitary gland cuts down production of the two hormones whose job it is to stimulate the growth of egg follicles in the ovary each month. As a result, the egg follicles secrete less of the female hormone estrogen (which normally builds up the lining of the uterus in preparation for the possible arrival of a fertilized egg), and the menstrual flow becomes scantier and less frequent. As time goes on, fewer egg follicles are stimulated and less estrogen is secreted until eventually the periods cease altogether.

But the "change of life" is not always such a smooth and well-regulated sequence of events. Hormone levels are temporarily thrown off balance, and may cause considerable variation in a woman's period pattern. In general, however, doctors give women these guidelines as to how their periods should occur at menopause: periods should just stop suddenly and not return; the gap between periods should gradually increase until they eventually stop; or the monthly flow should get less and less each time until it finally ceases altogether. Variations from these patterns are probably nothing to worry about, but they should always be reported to a doctor.

During menopause, the falling level of estrogen may cause other uncomfortable symptoms. The commonest of these are "hot flashes," in which a wave of heat sweeps over the body, usually from the breasts upward. Hot flashes usually last for only a few moments, but they may recur many times during the day. They are often triggered off by emotions, and may be followed by a wave of perspiration. Other distressing symptoms, which may or may not occur during menopause, include insomnia, fatigue, dizziness, heart palpitation, numbness in fingers and toes, headache (usually at the back of the head), itchiness (especially in the vaginal area), dryness of the vagina, skin changes, tingling sensations throughout the body, increased or diminished appetite, weight gain, and bouts of irritability and depression. While many of these symptoms are due to hormonal changes, emotional upset certainly plays its part in at least some of them. But any woman who finds that menopausal symptoms are becoming a handicap to her health and happiness should not hesitate to seek help from her doctor.

Is there any really effective treatment for menopausal symptoms?

Yes indeed! So much so, that no woman today need feel worried or apprehensive

133

about this phase of her life. For doctors have found that estrogen—usually prescribed in the form of tablets—can eliminate the physical symptoms of menopause. And the removal of physical discomfort will often help to lessen emotional difficulties, too. However, although thousands of women in America today are benefiting from estrogen treatment, medical opinion is split three ways on the subject of estrogen therapy. Some doctors advise women to take a daily estrogen tablet as soon as menopause begins—or even *before* it begins—and to continue taking estrogen for the rest of their lives. They maintain that estrogen not only does away with the problems of menopause, but also retards age changes in vaginal tissue, and prevents the development of heart disease and the thinning of bone structure which tends to affect women later in life (usually during their 60's). Other doctors recognize the value of estrogen in relieving hot flashes, excessive perspiration, and irregular periods, and in treating vaginal irritation, and will thus prescribe it on a temporary basis for women who suffer from these problems. They may also offer women mild sedatives if they are troubled by insomnia, or tranquilizers for mood changes, depression and irritability. But they disagree that lack of estrogen has any connection with heart disease or bone thinning, or that estrogen can keep a woman younger or more feminine. They say that the body continues to secrete a certain amount of estrogen long after menopause and that there is no need to supplement this. They suggest that the most effective way for women to combat any possibility of heart attack is to avoid overeating and to take sufficient exercise. Exercise will also help to prevent bone thinning, they say, and a further preventive measure is to ensure that your diet contains plenty of calcium.

Finally, a minority of doctors hold the view that menopause is a natural bodily process that should not be tampered with. They will not prescribe estrogen, but will confine their treatment to general reassur-ance and maybe a mild sedative.

This disagreement among doctors seems to leave the decision over estrogen largely up to women themselves. So what should you decide to do? Fortunately, a majority of doctors will prescribe estrogen, at least during menopause. And a leading U.S. gynecologist, having looked at the evidence on all sides of the medical profession, gives women this advice: "None of you should tolerate persistent hot flashes, or put up with vaginal atrophy [tissue changes causing soreness]. Insist that your doctor give you hormones for these disorders. If he refuses, find another doctor."

How long do menopausal symptoms last?

Symptoms, if present at all, may last only a few months or spread over periods of one to five years. They may begin months—or even years—before the ovaries cease functioning, and may continue for some time after the periods have ended. They vary greatly in intensity and frequency, but tend to become far less frequent as time goes by. It is impossible to predict accurately how any woman will react to menopause. But relatively few women are troubled by more than one or two symptoms, and these rarely last for more than a year.

Is there any way of telling when I will have my menopause?

The age at which menopause occurs varies greatly, and is impossible to forecast with any certainty. But women today seem to be reaching menopause increasingly later than in the past. A hundred years ago, the average age for menopause was 45. Nowadays, although some women may experience menopausal symptoms between their late 30's and mid-40's, the average age is 50 or over. A number of women do not reach menopause until 55, and in a few cases it may not be complete until age 60.

Heredity may have some part to play in determining when a woman will have her menopause, and there is also some evidence that, if a woman started having her periods early, she may have a late menopause—and vice-versa—but this is not always the case.

Will the menopause affect my sex life?

There is no medical reason why the "change of life" should alter a woman's sexual responsiveness in any way whatever. For the ovaries and the female hormones have nothing to do with sexual pleasure, and the external areas of a woman's body which respond to sexual stimulation are not affected by the menopause. In a few women the vagina may become more easily irritated after menopause, making intercourse painful. But this can be easily and rapidly put right by the application of a cream that contains estrogen, obtainable from the doctor.

Many women find that their sexual desire actually increases after menopause. When there is no longer any fear of pregnancy, a woman may become more spontaneous and relaxed in her lovemaking, so that the post-menopause years are the happiest of her marriage. Some women continue to enjoy a full sex life well into old age, while others find that their sexual needs gradually diminish. A lot seems to depend on a couple's general level of activity, health, and their previous sex life. Research has shown that 7 out of 10 couples are sexually active after age 60, and some healthy couples continue until age 90.

Why do some women get fatter at menopause?

Doctors agree that hormone readjustment is rarely the only reason for weight gain at menopause. However, decreasing amounts of estrogen in the body may be linked with a decrease in energy output, which means that the body needs less food to carry out its activities. So, if a women continues to eat the same amount of food as she has always done, she will get fatter. Sometimes, a woman may eat more than she used to, or just care less about her diet, because she is feeling low. But, in general, doctors blame the fact that women at this time of life, when the family is grown up, are often less active.

Whatever the reason for weight gain, it can and should be corrected for the sake of a woman's health as well as her morale. Doctors advise women to watch what they eat during and after menopause—plenty of protein and less carbohydrates is, as always, the rule—and to take regular exercise.

Is it possible for a woman to become pregnant even after her periods cease?

Yes, it is. Unfortunately there is no way of telling how long a woman remains fertile after the end of menstruation. And there are records of women who have conceived after the apparent completion of their menopause. More common, however, are the "change of life" babies who are conceived during, rather than after, menopause. For, while the periods may become infrequent for several years during the "change of life," the ovaries continue to produce some eggs. Quite a number of women between the ages of 50 and 55 have given birth to normal, healthy babies and the oldest woman on record to have become a mother was 57 years and 4 months old when her baby daughter was born. However, it is very unlikely that a woman will become pregnant later than a year after her last period, although some doctors advise women who do not want a baby at this age to continue practicing birth control for two years after the end of menstruation.

Is bleeding after the menopause always an abnormal symptom?

Once the periods seem to have stopped for good and all—and definitely if they have been absent for about a year—bleeding should never return. And any bleeding, however scanty, which occurs after the menopause must be investigated by a doctor without delay. The bleeding may be due to any number of minor causes, but it could be a sign of more serious disease. So never be tempted to wait and see if the bleeding recurs, but take this problem to your doctor as soon as you can.

Growing Older

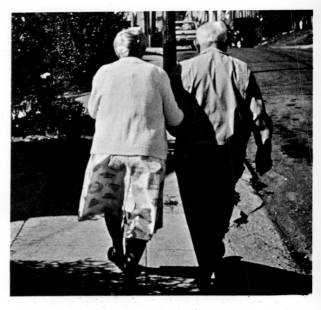

Why Do We Grow Old?

Medical scientists are divided on this question, and each group has its own favored theories. One group takes the general position that aging is caused by the accumulated effects of living: illness and injuries, over-eating, poor nutrition, too much tobacco and alcohol, too little exercise, and too much stress. They also hold that climatic conditions, and possibly radiation, induce aging. They support their arguments by pointing out that, since we have learned to control some of these conditions, people do live longer. In the 1700's, for example, a woman was lucky if she lived much beyond the age of 30; at the beginning of this century a woman's expected life span was only 48 years but today's average woman can expect to live until at least age 75.

Another group of scientists recognize that, while the way we live has much to do with aging, the real cause lies deeper in the cells. Cells in some tissues of a newborn baby are never renewed throughout life. And certain parts of the body—notably the blood vessels—begin to show age changes in quite young children. But, in the main, the human body actually *increases* its vigor and resistance for the first years of life, reaching a peak at age 12. If we could only stay as vigorous as we are at the age of 12, we should probably live to the age of 700. In the teens and twenties, things run along pretty smoothly. But about age 30 or so, cell functions begin to change. Some say that this is due to an accumulation of poisons in the cells. Others claim that the cells either "forget" how to renew themselves or follow the wrong instructions. And yet another group claims that aging results from

a change in the proteins which are the basic building blocks of life.

Any one, or all, of these factors may be the real cause of aging. We still do not know. But with more than 600 research teams working on the problem in the United States alone, the answers may not be long in coming.

How close are we to finding ways of slowing down the aging process and increasing life expectancy?

Although scientists have yet to discover exactly what causes aging, each passing year brings more and more evidence that it *is* possible to increase our life span, to stay young longer, and even to correct signs of aging that may already have begun to show.

As long as 30 years ago, Dr. Clive McCay of Cornell University doubled the lifespan of rats simply by cutting down the calories in their diet. Since then, other researchers, working on the theory that overeating hastens aging, have found that mice can be made to live twice as long as usual by eating normally for two days out of three and starving on the third day.

Another approach to the problem of aging has come through experiments with hormone treatment. In the 1960's, biologist Carroll Williams of Harvard University discovered a hormone that seemed to possess amazing powers of rejuvenation. This hormone, which comes from the brains of certain insects, was found to halt the aging process in animals quite dramatically.

Promising results have also been achieved by the use of chemicals. A drug which is widely used as a preservative in food has been found to increase the lifespan of mice by nearly 50 per cent.

Yet another approach has resulted from the development of transplant surgery. Many of the changes that come with age resemble changes that occur when the body reacts against a foreign graft. And some scientists have managed to increase the lifespan of mice with drugs that suppress graft rejection.

Up to now, none of these methods has been tried out on men and women, because this would have meant waiting perhaps 50 or 60 years of a person's life to judge the results. But it should soon be possible to measure aging over a short period—maybe 3 or 4 years—and see whether drugs or nutrition make any difference. Once such experiments start—and if they work—experts forecast that there could well be a 30 per cent increase in vigorous life by the year 2000.

Do women age faster than men?

The onset of aging—generally put at about age 30—is exactly the same for men and women. And the signs of aging seem to follow much the same pattern in both sexes. The one main difference is that, while men apparently retain their fertility until their 80's, or even 90's, a woman's fertility ends, on average, some time between ages 45 and 55. The change of life does not in itself produce signs of aging. But because, after menopause, women may appear to age faster than men, some doctors believe that lack of estrogen (which is no longer secreted by the ovaries after the menopause) may contribute to some of the more obvious signs of aging, such as wrinkled or less supple skin. Other doctors disagree. They point out that, although doses of estrogen keep vaginal tissues supple, estrogen cannot prevent or even slow down aging.

Some doctors hold the view that women age more quickly than men because the complex functioning of a woman's reprodutvie system makes greater demands on her body as a whole. Others disagree, saying that women are a good deal tougher than men, as evidenced by the fact that they live, on average, six years longer. Yet others believe that women simply *do not* age faster than men. They point out that no two people of either sex age at the same rate. Many young men and women look and behave as if they were already middle-aged; others remain young and active well into old age. The issue will probably only be solved when scientists uncover the secret of aging itself.

Can long life be inherited?

It is generally recognized that a person whose parents and grandparents had long lives stands a greater chance of living to a ripe old age. But this is not always the case. The aging process is almost always complicated by disease, and this makes it very hard to draw accurate comparisons between generations. So it's best not to count on inheriting a long life. Let's just be thankful that modern medicine can offer us a far better chance of living to a healthy old age than at any time in the past.

What is the greatest age to which anyone has ever lived?

The oldest person ever recorded was a Russian, Shirali Mislimov, who died in 1966, allegedly aged 160. He was said to have fathered children up until his 130th year. But his claim is discounted by doctors for lack of proof of his date of birth. The oldest authenticated record for long life to date goes to Canadian Pierre Joubert, who lived to the age of 115.

To most of us, life probably seems all too short. But we are still the longest lived of all mammals. Our nearest rivals are elephants, who may live to the age of 70. But the record for old age in the animal kingdom is held by tortoises that lived 150 years.

Things That Go Wrong

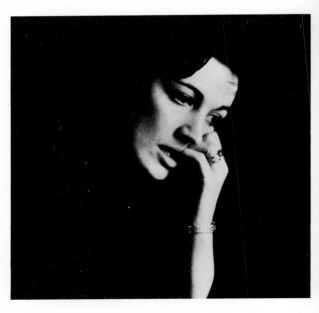

What is the cause of cystitis, and can it be easily cured?

Cystitis, a painful and distressing infection of the bladder, is usually caused by germs that get into the *urethra* (the tube from the bladder to the outside). It is one of the most widespread ailments. And it is five times commoner in women than in men. This is because a woman has a shorter urethra than a man, and bacteria can reach her bladder more easily. A certain amount of bacteria may enter the urethra as a matter of course, but they are usually killed off by the bladder. Occasionally, however, the bladder fails to defeat these germs. Infection may thus occur at any time, but is especially common in the early weeks of marriage (so-called "honeymoon cystitis"), during pregnancy, or just after childbirth. Doctors believe that "honeymoon cystitis" occurs because the movement of the penis against the urethra during intercourse stimulates the growth of the bacteria. Childbirth may have the same effect, and in pregnancy, there is an increased tendency to urine infection. The symptoms of cystitis are unmistakable. It is extremely painful to urinate—increasingly so as the bladder is emptied—and the urine may feel scalding. Yet the desire to urinate becomes more and more frequent. The infection may also cause pain in the lower abdomen and between the legs. And in cases in which the infection affects the kidney, too, backache, fever, and chills may develop. Fortunately, cystitis can be easily treated. Your doctor will probably send your urine sample to a laboratory. This is because many different types of bacteria can cause cystitis, and treatment will depend on which bacteria is found in your case. Before the lab report gets back, the doctor may meantime prescribe pills to relieve the discomfort. He may also suggest that you go to bed for a few days, and advise you to drink about two quarts of fluid a day for two or three days, increasing the amount to as many as three or four quarts every 24 hours. The fluid intake should be of any non-alcoholic drink, containing plenty of water. But too much tea or coffee, which may overstimulate the bladder, should be avoided. So much liquid will, of course, make you urinate more; but it will also dilute the urine and, together with the pills, will ease the pain. The symptoms usually disappear within a few days of treatment, and the infection usually clears up completely in about two weeks.

It's always a good idea to keep a note of the drug that controls cystitis for you. And another tip for women prone to cystitis is to make a habit of going to the bathroom within about 10 minutes after intercourse.

What causes vaginal discharge and itching, and how are they treated?

These symptoms, alone or together, are the commonest problems of women. Fortunately, these symptoms are rarely caused by a serious disease, and are easy to cure. In fact, discharges alone seldom require treatment.

138

All women have some discharge from the vagina. This is natural and necessary for health—the result of secretions that help to cleanse the vagina and keep it comfortably moist. Also, the female hormones produced during the menstrual cycle cause the cervix (the opening of the uterus) to secrete a small amount of sticky substance. Increased secretion of this kind may also occur in women taking the contraceptive pill. Finally, a certain amount of fluid normally seeps through the wall of the vagina and this increases during sexual excitement, or at times of sexual frustration, illness, worry, or emotional upset. Secretions thus vary at different times and from one woman to another. However, if the amount of discharge is really annoying, it is best to see the doctor, who may take a sample for examination under a microscope.

Vaginal itching, plus discharge, in and around the vagina are usually due to one of two main kinds of infection. The more common one is caused by a minute organism called *trichomonas*, which exists in the vagina of one in three women, and in the penis of many men. The organisms usually do not cause any symptoms, but in some women— for reasons unknown—they can cause severe itching and sometimes a frothy discharge. In this case, a doctor may take a vaginal specimen for laboratory examination, and will probably prescribe pessaries and pills. The husband must also take the pills, for he may harbor trichomonas without knowing it, and this is an infection that can be passed back and forth during intercourse. Symptoms usually go after a few days of treatment, and most cases are cured within a few weeks. The other main cause of an itchy vagina is a fungus infection, sometimes called "thrush". This is caused by a fungus that gets into the vagina and starts growing there. It can happen to any woman at any time, but is more common in pregnant women and diabetics. The latter have more sugar in the vaginal wall—just what this fungus likes best. Fungal infection causes a sudden intolerable itch and often a heavy discharge. It is almost im-

possible to resist scratching. As a result, the whole area may become sore, and urination painful. The infection may also give the husband an itchy penis. Once again, the doctor will first take a specimen for microscopic examination, and will probably prescribe pills to be inserted into the vagina, ointment for external use by both husband and wife, and possibly drugs. This treatment is effective and quick. In persistent cases, a change of drug—together with sterilization of bath, toilet, and towels—will usually do the trick.

My daughter is only 10 years old, and has already had her first period. Is this normal?

Girls today are starting their periods earlier than ever before, so it may be quite normal to begin as early as 10. In most cases, it only means that the glandular activity controlling the menstrual cycle has started functioning a bit sooner than usual. It is very important to reassure your daughter that all is well, and not to show alarm yourself. But, to ease your mind further, it is best to consult your doctor. He can make some routine tests to rule out the unlikely possibility of anything other than natural development being the cause.

Is occasional involuntary urination a sign of disease and is there a cure for it?

Doctors call this problem "stress incontinence". It usually occurs when coughing, sneezing, laughing, or straining in some way. It happens because the muscles that support the bladder and the vagina have been stretched or weakened. In mild cases, no treatment is needed beyond some simple exercises to strengthen the muscles. In really troublesome cases, which may be accompanied by a "bearing down" feeling in the abdomen or vagina, or a lump protruding from the vagina, an operation may be necessary. A doctor, will, of course, be able to recommend the best treatment.

Should you always urinate in a straight stream? And if the stream is not

straight, is this a sign of something wrong?

It is quite common to notice variations in the stream when passing water. Sometimes pubic hair may divert the stream. But usually variations are due to slight pressure on the bladder from the uterus which lies just above it. This is most likely to occur before a period or during pregnancy, and it is certainly nothing to worry about.

Is it normal for one breast to be larger than the other?

It certainly is. In fact, it is extremely rare for both breasts to be exactly the same size. The variation is usually only slight, although it can be quite pronounced and still be normal.

What causes inverted nipples and are they dangerous?

While a baby is developing in the womb, its nipples remain inverted, or turned inward, until a few weeks before it is born—and sometimes the nipples simply fail to pop out. They are not dangerous, and only need treatment if they do not come out during pregnancy to enable breast feeding. A few stubborn cases may not respond to treatment, but inverted nipples do not affect a women's health in any way.

What should I know about lumps in the breast?

Breasts naturally undergo a certain amount of change during the menstrual cycle, and just before a period, may become tender or sore and a bit lumpy, particularly in the upper and outer areas. If a woman examines her breasts at this time, she may be able to feel one or two definite lumps, but she shouldn't worry. Usually, when the period starts, the lumps disappear. Other women may have lumps in their breasts most of the time. The lumps vary in size, number, and location, but usually affect both breasts. Sometimes they go unnoticed, but they may cause occasional tenderness or pain, especially before a period. They may also cause discomfort for several months and then disappear for quite a long time. This condi-

tion, which is known as *chronic mastitis*, affects about 7 in 100 women at some time in their lives, but usually disappears after menopause. Its cause is unknown, although some doctors believe that hormonal imbalance is responsible, and may prescribe hormones as treatment. If a lump is particularly large or troublesome, a small operation may be performed to extract fluid from its inside and make it disperse. But if there is any doubt at all about the cause of the lumps, the doctor is bound to advise that they be removed and checked for possible malignancy.

What is the most accurate way of detecting breast cancer?

Since the chance of completely curing breast cancer is increased by early diagnosis, many doctors advocate self-examination by women (see page 118). If a doctor finds a lump in the breast, he may suggest X-ray examination (known as *mammography*) before deciding whether the lump should be taken out for examination in the laboratory. But a new method is now being developed that may enable cancer of the breast to be detected *before* there are any obvious symptoms. This is called *thermography* and it works by measuring heat rays in the breast. Cancer produces excess heat, which can be recorded by electronic patterns and made into colored photographs, or *thermograms*. These thermograms will also show up benign lumps, and other conditions that effect the breast, such as abcess, pregnancy, or even the contraceptive pill. It is hoped that thermography will be perfected in only a few more years.

What is a retroverted uterus? Is it dangerous?

Many women have a retroverted uterus and, in most cases, it is nothing to worry about. It simply means that the uterus is tilted backward toward the spine, instead of lying bent forward toward the stomach wall. About 10 per cent of women are born with a retroverted uterus. Others may develop one after childbirth, when the ligaments that support the uterus have been stretched. A retroverted uterus is merely a minor variation from the normal, and does not affect a women's functioning in the slightest.

What is a D and C operation?

A "D and C" is a surgical examination of the uterus, used to diagnose the cause of changes in a woman's bleeding pattern or other pelvic symptoms. This is one of the commonest of all operations, and sometimes is enough in itself to put matters right. D and C stands for dilation and curettage, because it involves dilating the cervix and using a curette to remove part of the uterine lining for laboratory examination. At the same time, the doctor can examine the uterus itself to check the Fallopian tubes and ovaries. A "D and C" is also done after a miscarriage to make sure that nothing is left in the uterus, and as a precautionary measure if bleeding occurs after menopause. The operation is a minor one that only takes a few minutes. Usually the patient spends no more than a day or two in the hospital. After leaving the hospital, most women can return to their normal routine at once. Menstrual periods may take a while to settle down, but this is perfectly normal.

What is a fibroid tumor, and is it related to cancer?

Fibroid tumors are growths that develop in the uterus. They occur in more than 20 per cent of all women, and they have nothing to do with cancer. No one knows what causes fibroids, which may remain quite small and insignificant or slowly grow until they are as large as a grapefruit. In many cases they cause no symptoms at all. But some women may feel a fibroid as a lump in the abdomen and, in certain cases, it may cause heavy or irregular periods. Fibroids can easily be diagnosed by a simple pelvic examination. Many require no treatment at all. But if one is causing troublesome symptoms, an operation may be needed to remove it.

What exactly is a hysterectomy?
Will this operation affect my sex life?

A hysterectomy—the removal of the uterus—is one of the operations women fear most. Many regard the uterus as an essential part of womanhood and worry that its removal will have a serious effect, not only on sexuality, but also on general well-being. This is not at all the case. The uterus has only one purpose—to carry a baby for nine months. Likewise, the uterine lining that is shed each month in menstruation, is built up for one reason only—to prepare for a possible pregnancy. The uterus has nothing whatsoever to do with sexual pleasure. And stopping the monthly periods by removing the uterus simply means that no lining is there to be disposed of. The only after effect of a hysterectomy is that the woman has no more periods, and she can no longer become pregnant. It is not true that cancer is the main reason for performing a hysterectomy. In fact, cancer is seldom the reason.

The operation itself may be done through an abdominal incision or through the vagina, in which case it leaves no scar. Usually, only the uterus is removed. But in some cases, it may be necessary to take out one or both ovaries and the Fallopian tubes. Then the doctor will prescribe estrogen pills to compensate for the loss of the ovarian hormones. After the uterus is taken out, the vagina is cut at its uppermost end. This does not shorten the vagina, and the cut heals completely in about six to eight weeks. After that, sexual intercourse can be resumed safely and satisfactorily. Remember that the enjoyment of sex has nothing to do with the uterus and ovaries. Some women find that they enjoy sex more fully because they no longer fear an unwanted pregnancy. Most women can leave the hospital about a week or 10 days after the operation, and are able to go about their normal activities quite safely. But doctors advise taking it easy and getting plenty of rest for about two months. You should, of course, avoid any heavy lifting, stretching, and strenuous exercise, such as sports, for at least three months. If you have a job, you may be able to go back to work between one and three months after the operation, depending on the type of work you do.

Some General Questions

I have heard a lot about the unpleasant side effects of hormone pills. Am I right to be worried about taking hormones, and is anything yet known about their long-term effects?

Millions of women are now taking hormones, usually as contraceptive pills or to control the symptoms of menopause. Yet most women feel a sneaking anxiety about swallowing regular doses of hormones, especially over a long period of time. It is well-known that the birth control pill, in particular, does cause side effects—such as nausea, increased vaginal discharge, "spotting," weight gain, or mood changes—in some women. Very often these effects disappear after the first few months. Some of them can be dispelled by a change of pill or by other medical treatment. But some women should never use oral contraceptives because they have conditions which may cause severe side effects. And no woman should start to take the pill without first consulting her doctor.

One of the greatest fears about the pill is the increased risk of blood clotting. But doctors say that this risk is often exaggerated. According to medical evidence, one woman in 2,000 taking the pill may develop a blood clot in a vein, but if that woman were pregnant each year, her chance of developing a clot would be twice as high.

Some women are afraid that the use of hormones may cause them to grow excess facial hair. But this is a needless worry. Almost all hormones prescribed for women are female hormones, which could not possibly cause any such masculine characteristic.

As to long-term effects, women have now

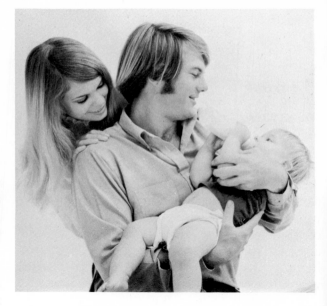

been taking the pill for 10 years or more, and no dangerous long-term effects have yet been found. The pill does not affect fertility. And there is no evidence that hormones cause cancer—in fact, hormones are sometimes used for the treatment of certain forms of cancer.

The contraceptive pill is a combination of synthetic estrogen and progesterone (the two hormones normally secreted by the ovaries). In treating menopause symptoms, only estrogen is given, and, in this case, many doctors prescribe natural, rather than synthetic, estrogens, which have virtually no side effects, and have never been shown to cause any trouble in the long term. But the one symptom that often bothers women taking the pill and women taking estrogen at menopause is a tendency to put on weight. In the case of the pill, this may just be a temporary weight gain of a few pounds in the week before their period. This is due to fluid retention, and disappears once the period is over. But it sometimes happens, both with certain types of contraceptive pill and with estrogens given at menopause, that the weight gain is a persistent problem. Doctors say that this is the result of excess fat being deposited in the tissues, plus the fact that women taking estrogen often tend to develop a heartier appetite. Alas, the only way to get rid of this extra weight is by dieting.

So, hormones do have their drawbacks, as well as their advantages. And although each woman must make her own decision about taking hormones, the best approach is to follow the advice of a doctor who knows your individual medical history.

How does a Pap smear work?

A Pap smear is a sample of cells from the cervix and the vagina which can be examined under a microscope. Named for Dr. Papanicolaou, who first developed them, Pap smears are used to detect cancer of the cervix long before it is visible in any other way and while it is 100 per cent curable.

Every day, cells in the uterus, cervix, and vagina are shed into the normal vaginal discharge. To collect some of these cells, the doctor simply inserts a narrow instrument into the vagina. This takes less than a minute to do and is completely painless. The sample is then fixed in alcohol and sent away to the laboratory. Because cells undergo a definite series of changes over a considerable period of time before becoming malignant, a Pap smear can pick up any abnormality at a very early stage—often years before cancer actually occurs. That is why it is so important for every woman to have a regular Pap smear once a year, or at the most two years. Then any changes in the cells will always be detected while there is plenty of time to treat them effectively.

Are there any medical reasons why a woman should, or should not, wear a bra?

Doctors agree that there is no reason why a woman with average-sized, firm breasts should wear a bra. And, they say, there is no evidence that a teenage girl needs a bra to keep her breasts from drooping later on. In fact, any woman can safely go without a bra throughout her life, except when she is pregnant, or if her breasts are large enough to feel uncomfortable without some support, because heavy breasts may stretch the supporting tissues. But, all in all, it is comfort that dictates choice in the bra debate.

Is there any evidence that it is better, from a woman's point of view, for her husband to be circumcised?

Apart from religious reasons, the points usually given in favor of circumcision are that it is more hygienic, improves sexual performance, and prevents cancer of the penis in men and cancer of the cervix in women. But most doctors agree that, provided little boys are taught how to keep their foreskin clean, there is no medical reason for circumcision. There is absolutely no difference between circumcised and uncircumcised men that might affect their sex lives. And, although cancer of the penis rarely occurs in circumcised men, this cancer seems to be related to lack of hygiene and will not affect uncircumcised men who are careful about personal cleanliness. A link between circumcision and cancer of the cervix has been suggested because this disease is less common among Jewish and Moslem women, who are married to circumcised men. Cancer of the cervix does seem to be related to sexual intercourse (nuns, for example, never get it), but research has produced no evidence that this cancer is caused by secretions found under the foreskin. Doctors who are against circumcision say that the foreskin has an important protective role to play. But, all in all, as far as anybody knows, there is no overriding medical reason for or against circumcision.

How many eggs does a woman have in her ovaries?

A woman is born with a lifetime's supply of 200,000 to 400,000 eggs inside her ovaries. But many of these disintegrate during the first years of her life, and by the time she is 12 or 13 only about 10,000 remain. Of these, a mere 400 or so will escape from the ovaries as mature eggs, ready to be fertilized. And when egg and sperm finally unite to create new life, the egg is probably at least 20—possibly as much as 40—years old.

143

For Your Bookshelf

Everywoman
A Gynecological Guide for Life by Derek Llewellyn-Jones, M.D., Taplinger Publishing Co. Inc. (New York: 1971); Faber & Faber Ltd. (London: 1971)

On Being A Woman
by W. Gifford-Jones, M.D., University of Toronto Press and Thomas Nelson & Sons (New York: 1971); William Heinemann Medical Books Ltd. (London: 1971)

Feminine Forever
by Robert A. Wilson, M.D., M. Evans & Co. Inc. (New York: 1966); Pocket Book edition, Simon & Schuster, Inc. (New York: 1968)

Let's Eat Right to Keep Fit
by Adelle Davis, Harcourt, Brace Jovanich, Inc. (New York: 1954, 1970); George Allen & Unwin Ltd. (London: 1971)

The Seven Ages of Woman
by Elizabeth Parker, M.D., The Johns Hopkins Press (Baltimore: 1960)

Let's Get Well
by Adelle Davis, Harcourt, Brace Jovanich Inc. (New York: 1952, 1970); George Allen & Unwin Ltd. (London: 1966)

This Slimming Business
by John Yudkin, The Macmillan Co. (New York: 1960); MacGibbon & Kee Ltd. (London: 1958, 1965)

Stay Young Longer
by Linda Clark, M.A., Pyramid Books, Inc. (New York: 1968, 1971)

The Body
by Anthony Smith, Walker & Co. (New York: 1968); George Allen & Unwin Ltd. (London; 1968)

Picture Credits